A **COMPLETE** GUIDE TO **PLEASURING** YOUR **PARTNER**

THE **SEX EDUCATION** YOU NEVER GOT

PAMELA HEPBURN FISK

NEWMAN SPRINGS PUBLISHING
320 Broad Street
Red Bank, NJ 07701

First originally published by Newman Springs Publishing 2021

ISBN 978-1-63881-333-0 (Paperback)
ISBN 978-1-63881-334-7 (Digital)

Printed in the United States of America

To Dinesh Kumar Viswanathan, my best male friend,
who inspired me to write this book

CONTENTS

Why I Wrote This Book 15

CHAPTER 1: Explanation of Contents of This Book 17
How This Book Addresses Its Targeted Audiences 17
Age Ranges and the Age of Consent 18
Cougars and Cubs 18
It's Not All about You: Selflessness 20
Mastery of Oral Sex 21

CHAPTER 2: It's Possible to Convert from a Taker to a Giver 24
Masterpiece Sex Life 24
Chemistry Is Important 25
Communication Is Crucial 25
Great Sex Creates Spiritual and Emotional Bonds 27
For Singletons: The Reality of Chemistry 27

CHAPTER 3: Beware of Players and Scammers 30
Sample Scammer Modus Operandi 30
Rejection: What Does It Feel Like? You Decide 31
Online Romance and Cybersex: What Could Possibly
Go Wrong? 32
Cybersex: What Exactly Is It? 33
More Statistics about Online Dating 37
Online Romance: Safe Sex 37
One Final Item Before We Begin: This Book Is a Buffet 38

CHAPTER 4: Introduction 39
Our Uptight Religious Culture 39
Shame and Societal Issues 40

Online Sexual Personality Tests 41
Sexual Repression in Other Countries and Cultures 42
The Results of Repression..............................42

CHAPTER 5: Adjusting Your Perspective 45
If You're Already Coupled Off 45
When It's Time for a Relationship, Get Tested for
COVID-19, HIV, and STDs..............................45
If You're on the Hunt 46
Role-Playing..............................46
But What If You're Not Especially Pretty or Handsome?..............47
Sexual Attractiveness: Does It Really Matter?..............................48
When Brains Win Out Over Looks..............................48

CHAPTER 6: How Things Work 50
Gaining Sexual Experience 50
Develop Your Sexual Skills 51
Inappropriate Sexual Behavior..............................53
Other Inappropriate Sexual Expression..............................53
Self-Consciousness/Embarrassment about Oral Sex..............54

CHAPTER 7: More about HIV and STDs 56
Body Far from Perfect? Accept It or Do Something about It...57
When the Opposite Is True: "Thick" Ladies Unite 57
Don't Wait Until You're Older to Come into Your
Own Sexually and Find Your G-Spot..............................58

CHAPTER 8: *Fifty Shades of Grey* Didn't Accomplish a
Damn Thing for Basic Sex..............................60
High School Sex Education Was Mostly Useless Too 61
Some of Us Are Just Too Serious, It's Time to Come
Out and Play..............................61

CHAPTER 9: A Good Sexual Partner Is Difficult to Find..............66
Oral Sex Worth Writing Home About..............................66
Penis Size..............................70
How to Measure Your Penis..............................71

CHAPTER 10: Gaining Experience with Cub-Cougar
Relationships 72
Figuring Out the Scene 72
16 Reasons Young Men Are Attracted to Older Women 73
Thoughts from a Seventy-Year-Old Woman about Oral Sex...74

CHAPTER 11: Sexual Preferences 76
Now for the Nuts and Bolts of Essential Basic Sexual
Knowledge 76
What Does It Mean to Be Straight/Heterosexual?.................76
Early Experiences 77
Sexual Urges of Children...78
What Does It Mean to Be Gay/Homosexual? 79
What Does It Mean to Be Bisexual? 83
What Does It Mean to Be Transgender? 84
What Does It Mean to Be Pansexual? 86
What Does It Mean to Be Polyamorous? 87
What about Nonbinary or Genderqueer? 88

CHAPTER 12: Sex Hormones 89
Estrogen 90
Testosterone 93
Progesterone...94

CHAPTER 13: Female Anatomy and Functions...............95
Breasts..95
Nipples...96
Pussy 96
Vulva..97
Vagina 98
Hymen..98
Clitoris...99
G-Spot 100
Orgasm 103
Cervix and Uterus 104
Fallopian Tubes 104

Fertilization 104
Menstrual Cycle 106

CHAPTER 14: Changing Sexual Urges (Female)......................108
Menopause..108
Decreased Sexual Desire 109
Decreased Arousal 112
Decreased Pleasure 112
Pain with Penetration 113
Thirteen Biggest Sex Drive Killers 113

CHAPTER 15: There Are Solutions 115
Benefits of Hormone Replacement Therapy (HRT) 115
Importance of Sex Hormones...............................116
Bioidentical Hormone Therapy.............................117

CHAPTER 16: More Solutions 122
Herbs and Supplements.......................................122
Natural Female Hormone Boosters........................122
Other Natural Solutions for Diminished Female
Sexual Interest 123
Acupuncture..124
Herbs for Female Sexual Enhancement..................124
What Else Can You Do to Improve Your Bedroom
Performance? 129
Special Workouts for Sexual Health......................129

CHAPTER 17: Male Anatomy and Functions.........................130
Penis..130
Ode to the Penis..130
Scrotum/Testicles 131
Nipples..131
Internal Male Genitalia 131
Prostate Gland...132
Symptoms of Prostate Problems 132
Additional Ways to Boost Libido.........................133
Male Orgasm 133

CHAPTER 18: Changing Sexual Urges (Male) 134
   Dealing with Male Sexual Dysfunction 134
   What Is Premature Ejaculation? 134
   What Is ED? 134
   Popular Commercial Drugs for Male Erectile Dysfunction...135
   Risk Factors and Side Effects 137
   Cheaper Sources for Drugs 137

CHAPTER 19: Alternatives to Pharmaceutical Drugs for ED.....140
   Acupuncture 140
   Acupressure 141
   Bioidentical Hormones 141
   Hypnosis 141
   What Role Does the Brain Play? 141

CHAPTER 20: Natural Herbal Aphrodisiacs 143
   Five Herbs to Help Erectile Dysfunction 143
   Product Warning: Natural May Not Be Safe 144

CHAPTER 21: Attracting a Partner 146
   Learn to Be Bold 146
   Banish That Shrinking Violet Part of Your Personality
   and Come Out into the Sunlight 146
   How and Where to Meet That Perfect Partner 146
   Caveat Emptor—Three of Them 147
   Flirting Online 147

CHAPTER 22: Online Dating 150

CHAPTER 23: Beyond Vanilla Sex 152
   Practices and Terms Used for Overweight, Heavy
   (Excuse Me, Fat) Women 153

CHAPTER 24: The Role of Porn 156
   Pornhub 156
   Personal Erotic Photography and Video 157
   Dressing Up 157

Props and Other Things 158
Massage Table and Virgin Coconut Oil Lube 158
Sexual Massage with Edging..159
Dressing the Set...160
Playing with Toys 160
Online Sex Toys 160
My Dildo and Vibrator Collection 161

CHAPTER 25: More Things Sexual 162
Anal Sex 162
Precum and Other "New" Things.......................................165
Masturbating (Female) 165
Masturbating (Male) 165
Masturbating on Video (Both Sexes) 166
Oral Sex and Gushing/Squirting 166
The Consistency of the Gush/Squirt 167
Oral Sex Information 168
Sitting on His Face..168

CHAPTER 26: Practice Safe Sex..170
HIV and Sexually Transmitted Diseases..............................170
HIV/AIDS 171
Other Sexually Transmitted Diseases (STDs)......................171

CHAPTER 27: Flirting with Photography and Video.................174
Attention, Men of All Ages, Gather Good
Photography to Help Attract a Partner 174
Photos for Your Profile: Dos and Don'ts 175
Erotic Photography and Video 176
The Pill-Swallowing Test 177
Ass Play 178
Prostate Orgasm 179
Breasts/Breast Man..180
Sexy Lingerie and Clothes 180
Muted Lighting..183
Music 183

CHAPTER 28: Communication Is the Key to Successful Sex 184
The Crucial Conversation about Sexual Preferences 184
The First Sex Questions That Many Men Ask 184
Questions for Ladies to Ask..186

CHAPTER 29: What to Discuss: Important Topics....................188
Types of Sex Preferred 188
Give Nothing but Pure Pleasure 189
Intercourse (the Polite Formal Way to Say Fucking) 191

CHAPTER 30: Preferred Hetero Sex Positions 192
Variations 194

CHAPTER 31: Now We're Getting Juicy................................196
What Have I Left Out? Foreplay 198

CHAPTER 32: Setting the Scene for Seduction..........................200
Preparations for Maximally Enjoyable Sexual Sessions..........200
Preparing Your Body 201
Pussy Smell: Natural or Carefully Washed 202
Pussy Soap...203
Before Sex 203
Men's Products 204
Choosing a Fragrance 204
Making Sense about Scents 205
Rules about Scents 205

CHAPTER 33: Women's Body Hair Removal or Not.................206
Female Genital Area 206
Men's Body Hair and Beards 207
More about Manscaping versus Shaving 207
Tips for Shaving Pubic Hair 208
Waxing and Chemical Hair Removers 208

CHAPTER 34: Other Physical Extras to Enhance Your
Encounters 209

Eyelashes 209
Notes about Tattoos and Piercings.....................209
Tattooed (Permanent) Makeup...........................210
More about Piercings: Tongue Piercing 210
Nipples..211
Nipple Piercing 211
Nipple Orgasms? Who Knew?..............................212
Genital Piercing (Female) 212
Genital Piercing (Male) 213

CHAPTER 35: Sexually Stimulating Getups 214

Feminine Clothing...214
Provocative Makeup for Women 215
What's Hot and Masculine 215
Mirrors..215
Do Alcohol and Drugs Enhance or Detract?.......215
Wineglasses 216

CHAPTER 36: Sensual Foods 217

The Best Timing for a Romantic Dinner.............217
Best Presex Food..218
Best Food for Sex Play.......................................218
Food Fit for a King and Queen 218
Types of Suitable Foods for a Sex Picnic in Bed ...218

CHAPTER 37: Sexual Lubricants...........................220

Coconut Oil (Heated Up) 220
Commercial Lubes 220
Author Reveal 221

CHAPTER 38: Sex Toys 222

Dildos 222
Vibrators 222
Butt Plugs 223

Lubes and Lotions 225
Massage..225
Happy Ending...226
Edging 226
Hair-Pulling 227
Spanking 227
B and D 227

CHAPTER 39: Light Bondage and Discipline 229
Soft Rope 229
Foot Fetish 229
Dominatrix 230
Submissive..231
Fingers 233
Fisting..233
Anal Sex 234

CHAPTER 40: The Penis.......................................235
More about Penis Sizes: Bigger Than Normal 236
Circumcised or Natural Foreskin...........................237
Oral Sex: Mind Over Matter 237
Blow Jobs (Sucking Cock) 238
Developing Oral Skills 238
Hand Job 238
To Swallow or Not, That's the Question 239
What to Look for in a Mate 239

Acknowledgments 241
Appendix 1: Is Pellet Hormone Therapy for Me? What
      You Should Know about Bioequivalent Hormones.243
Appendix 2: State Age Requirements (Age of Consent) 247
Appendix 3: Quiz 1 251
Appendix 4: Quiz 2..253
Appendix 5: A Cougar and Her Amazing Cub 255
Appendix 6: Big Red's BJ..259
Appendix 7: The Gay Paradox.................................265
Glossary 269

WHY I WROTE THIS BOOK

We've all had experience with that person who is just plain inept when it comes to sexual expression. Actually when we think about it, mostly everyone we've ever been to bed with is far from being that sexual dream we all hope for. Even that person with whom we were/are head over heels in love, with limited exceptions, just isn't/wasn't that great in bed. When we really think about it, many of us are chagrined to admit that we are committed/married to someone who is far from stellar in the sack.

Or worse, perhaps, we are painfully aware that we (you and/or I) are that person. What's even worse, we might be that total sexual dud and not even know it. In that case, you have probably been gifted this book as a broad and loving hint. Or perhaps we know that we aren't that sexual dream but just don't know how or where to start to change things to become better in bed. Sadly there are also those who are so darned selfish that they just don't feel like doing certain things sexually. Maybe because of the ick factor or maybe because they're just plain lazy. But don't give up. There's hope for all of us. And I mean all of us.

Relax, with this book as your main tool, I will help you to become much more knowledgeable and emotionally connected with your mate. Dare we suggest that you could become an expert at sexually pleasuring your partner? And as you read this book, you will undoubtedly decide to share what you're learning with that same person. Smooth move. Then the vibe between you is guaranteed to change. At a certain point, you will be instructed to do some surprising and exciting things. What about making a trip to a sex shop together to pick out the latest toys and some *lube*. The sex shop will be an assignment.

Ultimately your partner will become interested to sit down with this book as well, and soon, the sparks will not only start to fly in the bedroom, but you both will begin to achieve a deeper, more intimate connection and experience the many benefits that come with a truly mutually satisfying and deeply sexual relationship.

Is this a tall order? YES, IT IS, is my resounding answer. But soon, a measurable level of improvement in your sex lives IS ACHIEV-ABLE and within reach. Let's embark on this journey together. Just imagine yourself starting out on a golden brick road to the land of sexual excitement, a deeper connection, and newfound contentment.

It may come as a surprise that, in order to have a satisfying sexual relationship with your partner, you must first have one with—you guessed it, YOU. This book will equip you to have a healthier body, to develop a satisfying sexual relationship with yourself, and to maintain a strong *sex drive*. After all, you cannot share what you do not have.

CHAPTER 1
EXPLANATION
OF CONTENTS
OF THIS BOOK

How This Book Addresses Its Targeted Audiences

This is important, please read: This guide has been developed to provide information designed to answer sexually related questions of *straight (heterosexual)* men and women, *homosexual (gay)* men, homosexual *(lesbian)* women, *bisexual* men and women, *transgender* men and women, *pansexual* men and women, and last but not least, *polyamorous* men and women. While additional more esoteric *sexual orientations* have been identified, I will not venture beyond polyamorous for the purposes of this book, which is designed to address various issues and topics related to mutually satisfying sexual relationships, including a raft of information about sexual self-care and nutritional information.

To explain, the principal portion of this book begins with *heterosexual* (straight) sex, and yes, that section is the main focus. But please note that most health and nutrition issues that pertain to straight sex also pertain to other sexual orientations. After all, in many ways, we are alike. We differ according to our attraction to others. To illustrate, *HIV* and other sexually transmitted diseases *(STDs)* are addressed upfront, and please note that those diseases obviously apply to all sexual orientations. Please note that all words appearing in *italics* throughout the book are featured in the complete **glossary**.

That said, the array of general tips and information found in this book, except for the specific sexual practices of each sexual orientation, also applies to all. Many aspects of the psychology of a relationship, such as shared human emotions, include the desire to bond with your partner. There is so much more of value that pertains to all sexual relationships, not just the sexual orientations involved.

Age Ranges and the Age of Consent

You may wonder what ages we are focusing on with this book. As with the inclusiveness of the wide-ranging sexual orientations, we are concerned with every age that people could possibly have regular sex—from eighteen to eighty-plus. Although some states have established seventeen, and even sixteen, as the age of consent, we have chosen eighteen as the legal age for universally legal sexual activities. If consensual sex isn't part of your shtick, back off please. NO PERSON WILL BE REQUIRED OR FORCED TO ENGAGE IN SEXUAL ACTIVITY OR VIOLENCE OF ANY KIND.

Please note that the aspects of pleasuring your partner that need the most explanation, discussion, and analysis follow next.

Cougars and Cubs

When I was sixty-nine years old (2016–2017), I began my sexual exploration, aided by hormone replacement therapy (HRT), into the rich and exciting world of young men and older women. I had an amazing sexual experience with a twenty-year-old who I met on a cougar website. He was an amazingly skilled lover and clearly highly intelligent. He stayed overnight and was having such a great time, he hung around the next morning to chat for hours. Now that I am in my seventies, I have continued to meet younger men, and I've been learning quite a bit about the phenomenon of *cougars/cubs*. The most exciting descriptive information I have found is that these cubs are a devoted group to their often much-older cougar ladies, who derive their sexual satisfaction from younger men, their cubs. In fact, for some cubs, amazing age spreads fall somewhere between twenty to fifty years! According to liveabout.com, the "popular stereotype of a Cougar is a heterosexual white or black unmarried woman between the ages of 35 and 55."

Women in my age range (seventies) can certainly try a very young and willing guy but will probably find a simpler and easier experience, and probably more lasting, with someone in his forties, fifties, or sixties because of the higher levels of maturity. But wait. That said, there are always exceptions to declarations like that.

> To the feminist anthropologist, the recent attention shift toward Cougars can be explained by the increased scholastic and financial independence of women in the past few decades. Women of all ages and marital statuses are no longer financially tied to their male counterparts. With increased education and economic autonomy, women who were once thought of as romantically and sexually unavailable or off limits, have reentered the dating scene and are viewed by many as mature, romantic, exciting and experienced partners.[1]

An attractive forty-five-year-old guy who is into cougars shared with the author that he has regular sex with a woman in her eighties. Yes, and that woman's incredibly understanding and enlightened husband patiently waits in a separate part of the house until it's over. Whatever else you can say about it, that demonstrates extraordinary selflessness on the husband's part. I have a feeling that the husband was probably relieved that he was off the hook because she is a tad oversexed. He almost certainly couldn't manage her anymore.

---

[1] https://anthro2100.wordpress.com/2010/11/10/on-the-prowl-cougars-and-their-cubs/.

Cubs' ages vary greatly from late teens to sixty somethings. Many men in their forties and fifties, who have never married or had children and are living a long-time under-the-radar cub lifestyles, explain reasons for such attractions. For many cubs, age is only a number, and the idea of having encounters with much older cougars is actually extremely erotic and exciting. Who knew? A lot of people didn't know. At least until now they didn't know (more about cougars and their cubs on page 255).

"These older women are confident, sexually mature, they don't have inhibitions, they know what they like, and they know what they want," said Nancy D. O'Reilly, clinical psychologist, researcher, author and host of Voice America's radio program "Timeless WomenSpeak." Cougars are independent, career-oriented women who have a been-there-done-that attitude toward marriage and "don't need anyone to take care of them," she said. "They're looking for companionship, sexual contact, and someone good to talk to and spend time with. So be it if the relationship goes further."[2]

You'll enjoy exploring the short story "A Cougar and Her Amazing Cub" in the appendix on page 255.

It's Not All about You: Selflessness

What differentiates this book from the myriad books that have been published about sex? There are two things, actually. The first one is all about you. It may seem a bit like belly button gazing to focus on such things as self-care and healthy choices and the difficult process of finding a partner if you don't already have one. But without attending to those things, you wouldn't be properly equipped or have a personal starting point in your quest. What is this quest, you may ask, and the answer to that is to learn how to be totally and selflessly focused on your sexual partner in order to have the most mutually satisfying sex that is humanly possible to have. This sexual

---

[2] https://www.aarp.org/relationships/love-sex/info-07-2009/cougars-and-their-cubs.html.

destination couldn't be more attainable. Just pay attention and keep an open mind.

According to WebMD, "Research shows that couples who care about satisfying their partner—and who take joy from the other person's pleasure—are happier in the sack. This might mean having sex more often than you're used to, at different times than is normal for you, or acting out your partner's sexual fantasies."

Mastery of Oral Sex

And once you have figured all that out, the other essential ingredient is a mastery of *oral sex* to ensure the satisfaction of your partner. Of course, we're talking about straight heterosexual oral sex here, but the same principles apply with any sexual orientation. That's the piece that, if you learn absolutely nothing from this book, you must master completely, or you may as well just put this book back where you found it. Please refer to this area to discover all sorts of information about giving and receiving oral sex.

But wait. Even if you are just not into giving or receiving the pleasure of oral sex, there are various ways to overcome that aversion.* Don't stop reading about how to achieve the level of *selflessness* needed to truly sexually satisfy your partner.

Okay, so it's time to buckle down and concentrate on becoming the best in bed that you can possibly be. If your main goal in a sexual relationship is to pleasure your partner, it is certainly possible that during sex, you at least partially accomplish that goal while relieving your own *sexual tension*. In the bargain, you even achieve increased levels of personal satisfaction and intimacy with your partner.

But wait again. That, all by itself, is NOT ENOUGH. That pretty much describes many people's sexual relationships today. The key point of this book is: it's not all about you. For truly stupendous sex, it's much more about your partner. I mean, hello? This shouldn't be difficult to understand, and everyone, even the most inveterate sexual "takers" manage with effort to miraculously convert into "givers" if they apply the principles outlined in this book. And their sex life will improve.

*Ways to overcome an aversion to performing fellatio (please don't laugh): Practice on fruits and veggies. Using a dildo of normal scale and size, learn how to put on a condom. Lubricate. Lubricate. Lubricate with water-based product when you are using condoms. Sucking cock is intrinsically one of the sexiest acts on the planet.

Watch yourself in a mirror as you suck a dildo. Watch porn depicting fellatio. Allow yourself to actually become turned on to the idea of your performance of fellatio. It takes practice to become proficient at it. And once you do, you will probably crave it, knowing how much your partner enjoys it.

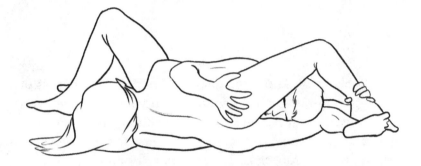

CHAPTER 2
IT'S POSSIBLE TO CONVERT FROM A TAKER TO A GIVER

Highlight: It's important to get this part. In the process of learning to focus specifically on your partner, you will even find yourself enjoying and getting into the giving part. That means you will learn to regularly give and receive oral sex, among other sexual acts, if these haven't been part of your repertoire until now. Once you get into it, it is hoped that you will crave to do these things for your partner just out of the pure joy of how your partner responds. This is the secret to selflessness. It's within reach of us all if we've truly taken the time to master selflessness.

Masterpiece Sex Life

It is crucial to be aware of the fact that reaching a deep understanding while focusing on your partner's satisfaction means several more important considerations yourself. That begins with adopting a heightened level of selflessness. Why? Because in that process, while you derive physical pleasure from the physical acts that you perform with that person, your truest satisfaction will be derived from the unselfish act of pleasuring your partner. It's as if your partner's body is the canvas, and you are the artist whose goal each time is to paint a masterpiece.

It is hoped that this book will equip you in every way possible to have the ultimate physical relationship by creating one masterpiece after another for what is to become your truly awesome sex life (the word *awesome* is so overused in our daily language, I promise that you won't find it reverberating throughout this book too often. I will use it sparingly to describe what I truly believe deserves to be labeled as truly awesome).

Chemistry Is Important

But I digress. There's actually more. We shouldn't leapfrog over the principles of sexual communication to begin or even jumpstart what was a great relationship. A great deal of personal satisfaction will also come from the spiritual and emotional bonds that you create while pleasuring your partner. And if the *chemistry* is right, you will also feel all kinds of loving feelings for that person. This will help move your relationship to the next level.

Communication Is Crucial

A sex therapy practice in Providence, Rhode Island, has published *Six Principles of Sexual Health.*[1] These are (1) consent; (2) nonexploitative; (3) protection from STIs, HIV, and pregnancy; (4) honesty; (5) shared values; and (6) mutual pleasure. It is recommended that you visit this site and read some excellent information and advice. It's almost like having a therapist and opening up about all that intimate stuff and going home with a pint of Ben and Jerry's and having a good cry. Seriously, you may end up deciding to go into counseling either alone or as a couple, which can both be a very good thing.

---

[1]   http://providencesextherapy.com/6-principles-of-sexual-health/.

A large part of pleasuring your partner includes communicating with that person in a highly personal and specific manner. In other words, say what you mean, and mean what you say. Don't bullshit. Period.

Below are six tips for communicating better in your relationship:[2]

1. Ask open-ended questions—Don't ask questions that are easy to answer with one word, but instead ask questions like, "How was your day?" That encourages opening up.
2. Pick up on nonverbal cues—Check out facial expressions: Are hands shaking? What's the body language? What about eye contact? Are they crossing their arms? What about the tone of voice?
3. Don't try to read their mind—If it isn't clear what they are feeling, ask. Don't say I'm fine when it's clear that you are not fine. Don't expect your partner to figure it out. Be direct. Don't be *passive-aggressive.*[3]
4. Conversations are a two-way street—This should be obvious.
5. Set aside time to talk—Obvious too.
6. Tell them what you need from them—Couldn't be more obvious.

There's a lot of useful information out there about communication. Self-help guru Tony Robbins offers ten ways to improve communication in a relationship.[4]

1. Commit to true connection
2. Identify your communication styles
3. Discover the six human needs

---

[2] www.Joinonelove.org.
[3] "5 Sneaky Behaviors That Are Actually Unhealthy," https://www.joinonelove.org/learn/5-sneaky-behaviors-actually-unhealthy/.
[4] https://www.tonyrobbins.com/ultimate-relationship-guide/key-communication-relationships/

4. Learn the three keys to passion and intimacy
5. Determine if your partner's needs are being met
6. Be honest and open
7. Be present in your relationship
8. Let things go
9. Break negative patterns
10. Start over

Great Sex Creates Spiritual and Emotional Bonds

Yes, that's why it feels so good when those bonds are being created. When sexual partners communicate on deeper levels and keep the happiness of their partner in the forefront, profound love has the impetus to result and grow. If you follow the directions in this book, you will learn about forming deeper connections with that person than you ever thought possible, because wonderful sex begets more wonderful sex, which, in turn, creates precious intimacy, which, in these days is a luxury to enjoy.

For Singletons: The Reality of Chemistry

For those who are not yet in an established couple: With only rare exceptions, that warm and fuzzy feeling that was just described won't be reciprocated with a new *hookup* (*one-night stand*), and that is a sad truth that is important to understand. Sometimes that fuzzy feeling never happens with certain partners, even those to whom we are so very attracted. It's just part of the language of love sometimes going haywire.

Yes, we have brought up the unavoidable factor called sexual chemistry. If a person just doesn't "feel you" for whatever reason, this is most probably due to the chemistry not being right between you. Unfortunately bad chemistry is pretty intractable, so you should probably learn to chalk things up to that and move on. Don't hang around trying to change things because usually they won't change.

The opposite of the concept of chemistry is true as well. If the chemistry is right, you will hit it off very well and have a great time together. But please be warned that you cannot possibly know whether your chemistry works unless you meet that person and actually spend time together. And when I say spend time together, I mean you could get a negative vibe almost immediately, or it may take longer to get to know the person. Please note that with the correct form of communication, a relationship that starts out badly can change completely and become quite wonderful. You both have to make a commitment to invest in the relationship. And then do it even if it requires therapy or marriage counseling.

When you meet, if the chemistry isn't right—perhaps it was the spinach in your teeth (only kidding)—or let's just keep it simple. You understand that it's over. But you want an explanation. This is it: Just chalk it up to chemistry and leave it to that, and don't take it personally. Otherwise you'll lose your stomach for the hunt and just give up trying to find someone who is really great for you and who appreciates everything about you.

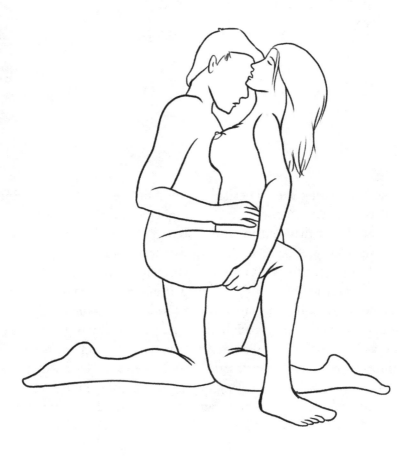

CHAPTER 3
BEWARE OF PLAYERS
AND SCAMMERS

Sometimes dating sites are called the ideal online matchmakers. But hold your horses. A romance that originates online may have you convinced that that person with whom you've made a *cyberconnection*, via Plenty of Fish[1] or Match or myriad other dating sites, is sexually attracted to or even in love with you. This is magical thinking and problematic right out of the gate and most often doomed to disappointment. If you don't meet in a safe place (restaurant, coffee shop, or bar) easily, it's possible that that person may be a scammer, who actually never plans or wants to meet you. Reckless behavior online can reap some pretty serious consequences. That's why there are standard warnings on dating sites against sending money because scammers ask for it. But many scammers have a modus operandi that is amazingly unimaginative.

Sample Scammer Modus Operandi

Scammers often have a "story" about where they are that they can't meet you until a future date. They claim to be on an offshore

---

[1] POF.com.

oil rig or some such remote place where they are effectively "stuck" for a while.

- Scammers are in love immediately, usually on day 1. They pounce on you, with long rambling often-romantic messages.
- They sometimes spend intervals during each day texting with you to get your attention and ply you with their carefully rehearsed story. That is often about how wonderful a person the scammer is, how age or distance are no barrier, how they care for a small child left behind when the wife died, and how the child is cared for at a special private school.
- Suddenly (at about week 3), there's a time when they might be able to meet you and begin your wonderful life together. But there's a hitch. Because of extenuating circumstances, the person needs cash for X, or they won't be able to travel to you. And you're the only one who can provide said money because suddenly, you are all important to the scammer.
- Unless you refuse (**which you must do**), you often will be asked for a quantity of cash or the use of a credit card or an iTunes card. I know, and that one is amazingly common. iTunes gift cards are popular because the gift card code can be exchanged for cash, so it has real value in the scammer's illicit world of scams and scammers.

Rejection: What Does It Feel Like? You Decide

I recall one situation when a man, whom I had met online, met me at a restaurant and clearly didn't immediately feel any sparks fly because the next thing I knew, he was headed for the exit. He rushed away so quickly that I had to pay the bill. As difficult as an experience like this may seem, you only need to recall the times when the chemistry didn't work for you with a particular person and just move on. Just say, "Next!" because it will prepare you to be open to the next person who comes along. Try not to get upset about these things when they happen. You cannot possibly hit it off with every single person you meet. As they say, there are *plenty of fish* in the sea. And you must believe that this is true. Because if you keep your relationship door wide open, someone special will come along if you know the way to attract him or her and what to look for in a mate.

> **Assignment 1: Men, if you are not particularly aggressive, learn to make the first move.**

Online Romance and Cybersex: What Could Possibly Go Wrong?

Most of us have heard about, or sometimes actually know, people who fell in love online, had a whirlwind romance, and got married and lived happily ever after. In fact, according to dating expert Hayley Matthews, "The way singles meet has drastically changed because of online dating." It's important to understand that with online dating, a lot of unique behavior goes with the territory.

Okay, here it is. Hold on to your hats. To add more to the challenges of dating, there is what I call *cybersex*. There are many men who only want cybersex, and, ladies, watch out, you might be online with a guy for hours, exchanging naughty photographs, before the guy finally *cums* while *masturbating* and then disappears, usually forever. I don't mean to sound callous, but as a rule, those guys aren't serious about finding either a mate or a date. It's also true that many online dating identities aren't even real people. While we must concede that we forge ahead even with doubts about online dating, we want to convey an important message that you have to be very careful indeed.

Gentlemen, if you frequent such popular online dating sites, don't be at all surprised when you encounter young ladies who ask for cash to get their hair, nails, eyelashes, and more done for your first date. There are those seeking a *sugar daddy* to take care of her and pay her bills. And of course, there are guys who would love to meet a woman who is financially comfortable and ask her to be his *sugar mama*. This actually happened to me! Online romance scammers literally spend hours every day seeking to separate you from your hard-earned money—another group entirely. You must educate yourself about all of this before you engage in online dating.

The Federal Trade Commission, Consumer Information website offers an informative article called "What You Need to Know About Romance Scams." A hair-raising statistic from that article is that people reported losing $201 million to romance scams in 2019. And romance scams were the most commonly reported fraud reported to the FTC in 2018–2019.[2]

> **Highlight: Online romance scammers often dedicate hours, days, and weeks to charming their potential victims.**

Cybersex: What Exactly Is It?

There are many men who, for various reasons, seek out sexual activities over the Internet. If you are dating online, you are probably experienced in that kind of *cybersex*. In my mind, cybersex is safe sex conducted online or on the telephone. That's what makes it safe—the very fact that you're online/on the phone instead of there in person. It starts with texting and maybe some racy photographs to juice things up and get them going.

Cybersex is defined on Google as "sexual arousal using computer technology, especially by wearing virtual reality equipment or by exchanging messages with another person via the Internet." I have to admit, though, to a complete lack of experience with virtual reality.

But let's talk some more about that elephant that's still sitting in the middle of our cyberworld for a while—scammers. It is a very simple rule: **don't be duped into transferring any amount of your money to anyone for any reason.** Stick to that rule, and you're good to go. This will be challenging. "Online-dating scammers are charm-

---

[2] https://www.consumer.ftc.gov/articles/what-you-need-know-about-romance-scams.

ing. You're not foolish if you fall for one—they are the most practiced chat-up artists the world has ever known."[3]

But do be careful when you meet someone online who claims to have fallen for you, before you've met in person. At best, that person is basically falling for an idea, instead of a person, when they fall in love before meeting the object of their ardor in the flesh. I mean, really, people, this is serious business here.

An article called "27 Online Dating Statistics & What They Mean for the Future of Dating," by Hayley Matthews, published online in June 2018,[4] is packed with great information.

> **Suggested online dating etiquette: Until you've met in person, always communicate only through the site (where you met them), and don't give out your full name, real address, e-mail address, or phone number until you feel absolutely sure you'll be completely safe.**

Most people take things comparatively slow, while scammers rush in. They will claim to have a "bond" with you immediately, you're their "soul mate," they've "never felt this way about anyone else before." They'll talk future, marriage, families—whatever you need or want to hear. Please be cynical *until you've met in person,* if the relationship has developed. If you want an external evaluation, show some of the messages to a couple of your trusted levelheaded friends and ask them to be gut-level honest. It's difficult to be objective when you have stars of love, sex, and romance glittering in your eyes.

> **Ladies, for obvious reasons, it is probably best to meet your dates for the first time at a simple nearby coffee shop or restaurant, rather than a bar or your home, for obvious reasons. And unless you are looking for a *hookup*, otherwise**

---

[3] "5 Ways to Spot an online-dating scammer," Readersdigest.co.uk.

[4] See appendix for article entitled "27 Online Dating Statistics & What They Mean for the Future of Dating," by Hayley Matthews, https://www.datingnews. com/industry-trends/online-dating-statistics-what-they-mean-for-future/.

known as a one-night stand, you should move slowly in the development of online relationships. Many cautious people choose to text or talk for quite a while before actually meeting in person. On the other hand, many also press for a meeting right away.

More statistics from that revealing article—and these may be deal breakers or outright scary—more than 50 percent of Americans lie on their *profile*, and over 60 percent of online daters are already in a relationship. And "one-third of women have sex on the first encounter with an online match, and four out of five women don't use *protection* on the first offline date."[5] That's scary stuff because it depicts irresponsible people engaging in high-risk behavior. Needless to say, this material is included because online dating is a very uncertain science.

---

[5] Ibid.

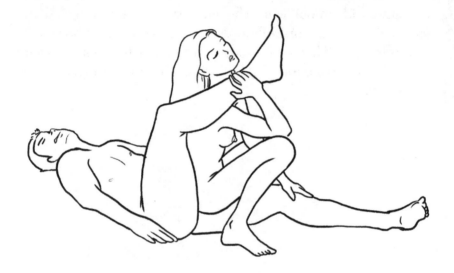

More Statistics about Online Dating

Other interesting points from this article are that 62 percent of dating app users are men and 38 percent are women. A healthy 59 percent of people think that online dating is a good way to meet people as opposed to 29 percent who feel that people who engage in online dating are desperate.

Yet a whopping one in five committed relationships begins online. And 17 percent of couples who married during the year 2017–2018 met on one of the over 2,500 dating sites in the US (there are over 8,000 sites throughout the world).

All of that said, remember, there's somebody for everybody. If you are currently alone and wishing for a mate, don't despair. If you follow the directions in this book, you have a good chance of finding a mutually satisfying relationship that endures. And if you're in a relationship that needs improvement, especially in the bedroom, this book should certainly help make things percolate again.

Online Romance: Safe Sex

"We are definitely seeing young people who don't practice *safe sex*," said Dr. Hansa Bhargava, WebMD medical editor and pediatrician based in Atlanta. "In a casual relationship, if a person feels like they 'know' the other person, they are less likely to practice protected sex" (more about this later, as well as discussion about STD and HIV testing being an essential part of every online dating app user's regular repertoire).

A British site called Online Dating Association offers a nifty guide to dating safely when the pandemic lockdown eases.[6] The link to this site is in the footnotes. The Date Safe area of that site is packed with good information.

---

[6] https://www.onlinedatingassociation.org.uk/date-safe/dating-safely-during-isolation-covid-19.html.

One Final Item Before We Begin: This Book Is a Buffet

Please note that this book is set up much like a buffet of information from which you are welcome and invited to pick and choose anything and everything that interests you. Just peruse the table of contents to decide which sections to read. If the subject matter in a particular chapter doesn't interest or apply to you, just move to the next.

For example, if you are not interested in information about herbal supplements that make you more sexual or virile, simply pass that section. But if you decide to do that, you might not do so well in a couple of entertaining quizzes that are designed to show your mastery of the voluminous amount of material being presented. It's up to you. After all, it's your book.

CHAPTER 4
INTRODUCTION

Our Uptight Religious Culture

Let's address some of the impediments to a great sex life that need to be overcome. First, there's *authoritarian religion*. The culture of the good old USA is rooted in Puritanism, a strict Christian religion that, much like today, rigorously prohibited sex between unmarried people. Sex was for *procreation* of babies by married people. Period. *Virginity* until marriage? Sacrosanct. Holy.

There was a time in history of widespread extremely uptight sexual restraint, when the top bedsheet for newlyweds had a slit in it for the insertion of the penis into the *vagina* of the wife, with no other skin-to-skin body contact allowed.

Another historic tradition that has persisted in many cultures is *wedding-night virginity testing*, when the bottom bedsheet is carefully examined for traces of blood to make sure that the bride remained a virgin until her wedding night, when her husband's role was to break her *hymen*. Otherwise the groom is stuck with "*damaged goods*," and in some cultures, the wife may be *disowned* by her family (amazingly plastic surgery to "*restore*" *the hymen* is popular even today).

While neither Puritanism nor Victorian morality continue to rule the marriage bed, religious control over people's sex lives has continued in some large sectors of our society until this day. Some Christian sects, such as Evangelical ones, are particularly strict, using the fear of damnation as a motivator to maintain one's innocence until marriage. Young girls participate in fancy ceremonies promising to keep their virginity intact until marriage. Often the fathers are involved in these ceremonies, a practice that seems particularly creepy to me because it's like a prom with Dad as your date. The main drawback of all of this is that individuals end up marrying each other without knowing if they are *sexually compatible*. Because of *social or religion-induced guilt*, these married couples awkwardly engage in a struggle to overcome inexperience and embarrassment while discovering each other's bodies as well as their own. It's a slippery slope, indeed.

> **News flash: Now is the time to disabuse yourself of any vestiges of sad puritanical ideas that sex is dirty and disgusting. In its purest state, sex is a God-given expression of selflessness and love. And probably more often, it's just a randy expression of intense horniness. And there's absolutely nothing wrong with that either.**

Shame and Societal Issues

Even today, in many American social settings, it simply isn't acceptable to express one's sexuality openly and honestly. As we grow up, many of us are taught that sex is forbidden territory. Children's natural urges to explore their bodies and masturbate are often discouraged firmly by parents and caregivers. Little babies who touch themselves are taught that that is naughty, and they are carefully instructed not to do it. And these attitudes continue into *puberty* and adulthood, at least at an unconscious level.

> **Gals, please buy various kinds and sizes of *condoms* and keep them in the bedside drawer and in your purse.**
>
> **Guys, buy condoms, keep them handy, and always use them. For safe oral sex with a female, dental dams are what you need for protection against HIV and sexually transmitted diseases (STDs).**

Boys wishing to look at "dirty" pictures of women and masturbate normally only do that in privacy when they won't get caught in the act. Girls discreetly stuff their shirts with socks to simulate breasts and quietly explore and play with themselves in front of a mirror, in the privacy of their bedrooms. The girls are very commonly trying out kissing, touching, and other sexy things with one another during sleepovers. These are all parts of *normal sexual development*. Virtually everyone has their versions to tell you about.

I know a woman who, about ten, got carried away experimenting and soaped up her *vulva* during her shower to the extent that it burned like crazy afterward. She learned a difficult lesson. She never did that again (oh all right, it was me). I'll never forget that burning. And I knew I couldn't tell anyone about it. I was clear about that. It was just too embarrassing. That's a sad commentary, isn't it? So now I get to tell the world about it in this book. Go figure.

Our society is still so uptight that even mothers wishing to breastfeed their infants in public are admonished to do it in private. A young woman who dresses in a sexy manner to arouse her man or to attract men in general is still called cheap or slutty in many parts of our society, when she is really only expressing both her femininity and her sexuality. The rape victim is told that she attracted the rapist with the clothes that she wore that fateful night. This atmosphere creates feelings of shame around sex and hang-ups about acting out our most natural instinctive sexual thoughts and fantasies.

Online Sexual Personality Tests

I invite you to not only give up the guilt but to embrace your sexuality and learn about your *sexual personality*. There are all kinds of online sexual tests to help you do this. A couple of recommended ones that illuminate your sexual personality are found in the Psych Central and Psychology Today sites (https://psychcentral.com/quizzes/sexuality-relationship-tests/ and https://www.psychologytoday.com/us/tests/relationships/sex-personality-test).

Sexual Repression in Other Countries and Cultures

The USA isn't the only country where shame surrounds the world of sexuality and its expression. Despite the fact that the famous ancient *Kama Sutra* philosophy of life and accompanying representation of sixty-four sexual acts originated there, East Indian society continues to repress the sexuality of its young people. In fact, Indian movies are finally allowed to depict kissing on the screen. So now Bollywood actors are not only kissing, they seem to be going crazy, showing all kinds of suggestive movements in their ubiquitous movie dance numbers, with everyone vigorously thrusting their hips in ways that are almost embarrassing caricatures of sexuality.

Other countries where excessive sexual repression is common and sex outside marriage is strictly illegal include the Muslim countries of Saudi Arabia, Afghanistan, Iran, Kuwait, Morocco, and United Arab Emirates, among others.[1] According to Wikipedia, "various cultures attempt to repress homosexual sexual expression. As of 2014, same-sex sexual acts are punishable by prison in 70 countries, and in five other countries and in parts of two others, homosexuality is punishable with the death penalty."[2]

The Results of Repression

It's important to recognize that there are many negative societal outcomes that result when our sexuality is repressed. An online article that illustrates this in perhaps its most extreme form is found in a blog by Dr. Christopher Ryan, sponsored by *Psychology Today*:

> **Nothing inspires murderous mayhem in human beings more reliably than sexual repression. Denied food, water, or freedom of movement, people will get desperate and some may lash out at what they perceive as the source of their problems, albeit in a weakened state. But if expression of sex-**

---

[1]   "Sexual Repression," Wikipedia.
[2]   "Where is it illegal to be gay?" retrieved July 29, 2019.

uality is thwarted, the human psyche tends to grow twisted into grotesque, enraged perversions of desire. Unfortunately, the distorted rage resulting from sexual repression rarely takes the form of rebellion against the people and institutions behind the repression. Instead, the rage is generally directed at helpless victims who are sacrificed to the sick gods of guilt, shame, and ignorant pride. [3]

Because of its downright harshness, that statement is a direct warning about the importance of the full and natural expression of human sexuality. It basically states that people should be able to experience their sexuality without guilt or unreasonable restrictions. Of course, that doesn't mean that people should be totally inappropriate in their sexual expression, which means there is a time and a place for everything. Some of the worst and most inappropriate sexual behavior includes *rape* and *pedophilia*. And *date rape*, often aided with drugs slipped into ladies' cocktails, is appallingly common.

---

[3]   https://www.psychologytoday.com/us/blog/sex-dawn/201004/sexual-repression.

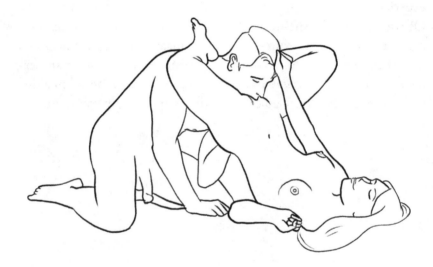

CHAPTER 5
ADJUSTING YOUR PERSPECTIVE

If You're Already Coupled Off

If you're in a couple, either married or in a committed long-term relationship, there is a reason that you are reading this book. Undoubtedly that reason is that something isn't quite right with your sexual relationship. Choose one: The sex just isn't great. The thrill is gone. You're just going through the motions nowadays. You're not getting enough/any sex. Major ingredients, like excitement, are missing from your relationship. There's no oral sex. Or only one of you performs oral sex. Sex is always the same/too predictable. Have I covered the gamut? Large portions of this book are for you and your partner. Knowledge is power.

When It's Time for a Relationship, Get Tested for COVID-19, HIV, and STDs

When you realize that you've been hanging around with your dog (or cat) much more than another human being, and that you haven't had sex in forever, perhaps it's time to get into a relationship. Perhaps, needless to say, COVID-19 testing and vaccination are the first steps before you do anything else. Of course, everyone should be vaccinated. See page 56 about HIV and STDs testing.

If You're on the Hunt

Maybe you're quite young and want to learn about great sex before you find a girlfriend or boyfriend. Or perhaps you're fresh out of a disappointing relationship. Or you've been "playing the field," and you'd like to settle down with one sexual partner, which, with the diseases that are going around, is a very wise choice. Or you're newly separated or divorced and painfully aware that your sexual relationship was nothing to write home about.

Or perhaps you've decided to become a cougar on the hunt for cubs. Or you've realized that you're attracted to older women, and it's time to become the cub that you were meant to be. Perhaps you're also a budding cub who realizes that he prefers "thick" (or voluptuous, curvy, or fat) women to those with a Barbie doll physicality. That is actually another fast-growing trend today. Yes, it is a real thing. Who knew?

Role-Playing

Instead, it might be that you've decided that you want to find someone who is willing to dress up and act a part in some serious supersexually charged *role-playing* activity. Many people find that to be extremely fun and satisfying. Some roles include the obvious: stepmom and naughty son, or the teacher and student, both of which require the son or student to be told what to do or be "punished."

To be really exciting, *role-playing* requires a rich imagination, along with a lack of self-consciousness or embarrassment. If it still feels just too weird, once you try to get over that weirdness, you may realize that it may not be for you. If you find the idea titillating, do some role-play. You'll never know if you like it if you don't try. What about dominatrix (dominant) and submissive? This is the activity that the *Fifty Shades* books and movie made so famous. Yes, we'll get into that too.

No matter what your situation, this book will give you the pointers you need to become the kind of sexual partner in your next alliance that will bring excitement and life to your relationship. The main thing I ask from you is an open mind. If you take the directions in this book to heart, I can almost guarantee that your next relationship will be the best you've ever had. Sexually. Emotionally. Physically. Yes, all of the above. How? When you understand that the desire to pleasure your partner is your main focus, your perspective changes, big-time.

But What If You're Not Especially Pretty or Handsome?

What should a person do if he/she isn't very physically attractive to another sexual partner? Well, this is challenging but not insurmountable. Don't give up. Welcome to the human race. The truth is that most of us are average in the looks department, which means we are far from hot. But there is a solution. Stick with us here because this will take a serious commitment on your part.

> **News flash: If you aren't graced with a handsome or pretty face and/or body, you'll need to compensate in other ways. You'll need to develop some serious skills. I am talking about sexual skills here—*fellatio* and *cunnilingus*.**

As they say, there is someone for everyone, which means that there is a sexual partner, and yes, even a great sexual partner out there, even for those who wouldn't win a beauty contest. This endeavor definitely requires extra effort. First, seek out people who are your aesthetic equals, meaning people who are in the same category as you are as far as looks are concerned.

You will undoubtedly find that many of those people have developed themselves in other and usually more valuable ways. For example, they may excel in the brains and educational achievement arenas. Or they may be stars in their field of work or other endeavors. Some people are great in sports. Others have particularly winning personalities or are especially amusing and enjoyable to be around.

Still others have *animal magnetism* despite their lack of physical looks, which has everything to do with self-confidence and poise. A fairly homely person with confidence and expertise in bed has two of the most crucial keys to sexual attractiveness right off the bat. Confidence and expertise often come with extensive experience, all of which are also considered important keys to sexual attractiveness.

Sexual Attractiveness: Does It Really Matter?

Let's face facts now; looks are no guarantee that someone is great in bed because he or she might be a complete jerk with even the greatest looks. This goes for both men and women. A gorgeous woman could be the world's biggest airhead or bitch and ruin the sexual moment every single time with her irritating voice. And there are handsome men who are so *narcissistic* that it seems that no one is perfect enough for them. Sometimes the best-looking people are insufferable because of their good looks. We all know that good-looking person who doesn't have one ounce of self-confidence. What horrible negative messages were conveyed to that person when he or she was growing up? Attractive people are often accused of being full of themselves. We've all met this kind of person. Or perhaps we are that person.

What are some other important keys to success in bed? The answer to this is *sexual attractiveness*. A few essential qualities of a person who has that sexual attractiveness include the willingness to be unselfish, adventurous, and have the ability to suspend the yuck factor (more about all that on pages 95 and 276).

When Brains Win Out Over Looks

In assessing what attracts you to others, you may realize that you are a *sapiophile* or *sapiosexual*, which are newly minted popular terms for a person who is both intelligent and sexually attracted to brainy people (these words are being used more all the time, especially in the online dating world). Looking for native intelligence in your mate is a less shallow way to be because merely insisting that your partner be physically attractive doesn't guarantee happiness at all. But if we are honest, it is fairly restrictive to look only for brainy people as well. But if you are brainy, it's probably a given that you wouldn't be attracted to someone who isn't somewhere in the same league. And vice versa. A potential mate that attracts us because of his or her animal magnetism can also be a great relationship but just on a different intellectual plane. You won't be discussing weighty matters of the world, but your sex life will be stellar.

CHAPTER 6
HOW THINGS WORK

Gaining Sexual Experience

How does one gain confidence and expertise? Where does that experience come from? Early sexual practice often colors every experience that comes later. With each sexual experience, a person learns more, as long as they keep trying new things and don't get caught in a rut of performing the same sex acts every time.

A couple who only engage in *missionary-style sex* when the guy on top *cums*, and then he climbs off and falls asleep is what I'm talking about here. It is time to diversify, people. It's time to learn how to do it right. Believe it or not, doing it right involves thinking of whether your partner had an *orgasm* and making sure that the session doesn't end until both of you have satisfying orgasms. This is key to true intimacy and is perhaps the most important ingredient of a loving relationship. It all boils down to selflessness. If your partner doesn't care, your relationship is probably headed for the rocks.

But how do we know if we're "doing it right"? Gauging from their partner's response is the best way to measure effectiveness of sexual techniques. Verbal forms of appreciation, including moans, work best. Remarks like "That was great!" work too. Communication is extremely important. Some people verbalize with *dirty talk*.

And then there's the desire for more sex. Regular sex. One to two times a week. More frequent sex. Are three to four times a week enough sex? Or are you exceedingly horny and want it every day, or sometimes more than that? I have a friend who either has relations with his wife or masturbates every single day, and often both. And he's in his early fifties, and they've been married for twenty-plus years. Is that "too much?" Trying to figure out how much is enough is an embarrassment of riches we all wish to have.

Develop Your Sexual Skills

If you've recognized that you aren't a star at attracting the opposite sex, don't just sit there feeling sorry for yourself. It is the time to develop yourself in other ways, not only educationally and/or in your career but sexually as well. If you are blessed with sizable *genitals* (man's penis or woman's ass and breasts), those may be of considerable help. If that is the case, and even if it isn't, you should definitely—no, you absolutely must—develop your sexual skills. This is the main point of this book about pleasuring your partner.

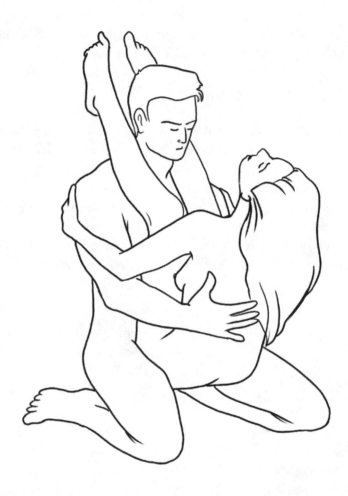

Inappropriate Sexual Behavior

What about a young lady and an older man? That doesn't bring a positive connotation with it, does it? To wit, the *#MeToo* generation of women who are increasingly willing to come out and share their stories of abuse by men who were trusted by those, including parents, who didn't know these men were sexual abusers.

Why is this so sensitive an issue for our society? Because a significant percentage of the population preys on younger people to satisfy their twisted sexual desires. And the victims are left with hang-ups and trust issues and PTSD for the rest of their lives. Many become alcoholics and/or addicts.

Young men are too often preyed upon by (yes, mostly heterosexual) *pedophiles* who threaten them with horrible kinds of retribution if they tell anyone about their abuse. Many of these pedophiles are in employment or volunteer situations where they, by their very positions, are often in direct contact with young people. These often include teachers, coaches, scout leaders, priests and ministers, even doctors. And sadly, parents, relatives and siblings, uncles, aunts, and cousins are pedophiles too, and prey on younger people, including family members.

To ensure that those individuals holding such positions are responsible and will not sexually prey upon young people, it is incumbent upon parents to check them out carefully and thoroughly before entrusting children to them. And because children are often threatened not to tell anyone, it's crucial that parents make clear that children should always feel comfortable telling a designated trusted adult.

Other Inappropriate Sexual Expression

Many small-town baby boomers remember fondly the times when they drank beer and made out and had sex in cars parked in secluded locations, like wooded areas in the countryside. In order to get some private time, this was a common way to spend a Saturday night. But almost inevitably, there would come the *tap, tap, tap* of the policeman's nightstick on the window that was fogged up from the couple being hot and bothered inside. Nothing but embarrassment ensued in these circumstances.

Children and adults caught masturbating and couples copulating or performing sex acts in public are definitely subject to both scorn and arrest. It's called exhibitionism. And while it may be titillating to attempt, those and other sexually charged behaviors in cars or outdoors where people may see you, those behaviors are best left to the indoors where privacy and free reign to do whatever your imagination dictates, within some basic boundaries, including making sure that no one gets hurt.

You may wonder why these warnings are appearing in a how-to type of sex book. It is simply because for virtually every healthy sex act, there is an unhealthy sex act. That is unfortunately how twisted some people can be. I'm talking about sexual impulses such as pedophilia. It's important to not only acknowledge this but to fight the spread of unhealthy sex by getting out of unhealthy sexual situations, developing our healthy sex drive, and having a great sex life.

Self-Consciousness/Embarrassment about Oral Sex

Then there's the person for whom many of the most acceptable normal sexual acts make them feel awkwardly self-conscious or embarrassed. A man who is self-conscious about the size or quality of his own *hard-on* isn't going to do so well in the bedroom. People who cannot perform what they feel may be "dirty" or "icky" acts on their partners are at a distinct disadvantage sexually.

They also put their partners at a grave disadvantage. Imagine being stuck with a sexual partner who finds any part of your body as a sort of no-man's-land that is doomed for the life of the relationship of being undiscovered and unexplored. And yes, this happens far too frequently. That is partially why this book was written.

Individuals who react to the performance of various sexual acts in these ways are limiting the full expression and experience of their own sexuality and cheating their partner out of theirs as well. This is the key problem in American sexual performance. People are often just too self-conscious or embarrassed to open themselves up to what are the most natural and awesome sexual expressions—*fellatio* and *cunnilingus* (more about these on pages 271, 270).

Often regarded as *taboo*, oral sex isn't actually banned in most countries. But people may also have sexual inhibitions about giving or receiving oral sex or may flatly refuse to engage in the practice.[1] There is much more to cum (pun intended) about these two major ingredients to successfully pleasuring your partner. You may wish to fasten your seat belt (see pages 189 and 274 for more on oral sex).

---

[1] https://en.wikipedia.org/wiki/Oral_sex.

CHAPTER 7
MORE ABOUT
HIV AND STDS

The CDC offers its website for the recommended HIV and STD tests one should get when you are sexually active.[1] STDs are sexually transmitted diseases.

Rule 1: Make sure you are disease free.

You can get HIV and STD testing at many places, such as the following. Run a search on Google for "local HIV and STDs testing." And name your location.

- Your health-care provider's office
- Health clinics or community health centers
- STD or sexual health clinics
- Your local health department
- Family planning clinics
- VA medical centers
- Substance abuse prevention or treatment programs

---

[1] https://www.cdc.gov/std/prevention/screeningreccs.htm.

Body Far from Perfect? Accept It or Do Something about It

Now it's time to take charge of those things we haven't been managing particularly well. Those men who have double chins and potbellies (you know who you are) may use that as an excuse not to do much more than wham bam, thank you, ma'am, in the bedroom. Believe it or not, that is defined online as sexual activity conducted roughly and quickly, without tenderness.[2] If you are in a relationship, half of your battle may already be won. Your woman probably accepts, or at least tolerates, your excess weight. And she may be equally heavy or out of shape. So now it's time for you both to buckle down to either lose the weight and learn how to satisfy your partner or keep things at the status quo, meaning you just continue to neglect to lose weight and just do your best to satisfy. But the former is preferable because your body needs to be in good shape to employ many intimate tricks.

And gals, many of whom have reached middle age sexually, or should we call it sexual maturity. Word salad aside, things just aren't the way they used to be. It's time to take control and jump-start your life. The time to begin is now. That, for what it's worth, is my rallying cry. The time to begin is now.

When the Opposite Is True: "Thick" Ladies Unite

Ironically we go from a fit woman back to a thick woman in the next breath. A woman who has a tummy and a large rear end and quite a bit of excess weight could comfort herself in knowing that there are actually men who prize a voluptuous woman. In fact, there is an entire segment of the population of younger men who actually love and pursue that rarified group they call older "thick" ladies as a generous segment of the cougar-cub phenomenon. This means curvy, voluptuous, or outright overweight, depending upon your mindset and level of self-honesty. Okay, okay. I'll say the word—*fat*

---

[2] *Oxford.*

When asked, these cubs might explain it this way, "Who wants a scrawny boney Barbie doll body?" If you're unfamiliar with this, I know what you're thinking, but this has truly become a thing. It can't be denied.

The point is that physical imperfections don't have to hold anyone back from enjoying a fully intimate sexual life. And if you really have a problem with it, get your butt in gear and exercise and eat less, diet and lose the weight, and get into shape. I won't be there to hold your hand through this process. Make a decision to just do it, as Nike would say.

Don't Wait Until You're Older to Come into Your Own Sexually and Find Your G-Spot

I know a woman in her seventies who waited until she was in her late sixties to blossom into a fully realized sexual being. To illustrate, she didn't know where her *G-spot* was until she reached her seventieth year, and a girlfriend told her about glass dildos that have ridges around them that are designed specifically to stimulate the G-spot. During all those years before this crucial discovery, she had thought that that illusive and mysterious place for amazing orgasms was somewhere deep in the recesses of her vagina, as if it were some truly unfathomable treasure. Well, when she used the glass dildo for the first few times, she was gobsmacked. The ridges in the dildo actually stimulated the place that ended out to be her G-spot. So that's where it is (more, including the G-spot location, on pages 100 and 271).

> **Rule 2: Have oral sex with your partner at least once a week.**

Another friend in her seventies looks and acts quite a bit younger than her age partially because of what must have been highly favorable genetics, which prevented the onset of wrinkled skin, and also because she was just an open and direct person who wasn't afraid of what people would think of her if she had some hot sex with younger men, sometimes even ridiculously younger men. On occasion, she even shares some of the hotter naked photos with the girls at the condo pool.

Rule 3: Men with a small or just an average penis can make up for it with great oral sex techniques. Think about it.

CHAPTER 8
FIFTY SHADES OF GREY DIDN'T ACCOMPLISH A DAMN THING FOR BASIC SEX

If we think about it for a moment, the lessons we learned from *Fifty Shades of Grey* didn't go very far in the area of *basic sex 101* and the truly necessary ingredients to provide pure and pain-free pleasure to your partner. The emphasis of that series of books, and the movies that followed, stressed inflicting pain, manipulation, hostility, suffering, domination, and mind games as tools for seduction and relationship building. I'm sorry, but I just don't buy it as a viable lifestyle. So that, in a fat nutshell, is my opinion. All of that said, the author is raking in the dough on the books, movies, and sex toys galore of the *Fifty Shades* phenomenon. I find it ironic that S and M is what's being offered up as a way of being in a time when tenderness and gentleness are needed more than anything. It seems that we all have some version of *PTSD*.

While it did increase interest in *BDSM*, most of us came away from that entire *Fifty Shades* phenomenon with little more than a few usable pointers for our own experiences in the bedroom. What about covering the finer points of seduction? Oral sex? Preparation for hot sex? What about just plain kind and unselfish sex where the urges, needs, and preferences of your partner are all foremost? What a concept. Those are the subjects we all need to master if we want a great sex life and want to provide our partner with great sexual experiences. And those subjects are all covered in this book. You will find that reading and making this book the center of a successful sex life is a main goal for a thriving erotic relationship. That is because knowledge is power.

High School Sex Education Was Mostly Useless Too

As those of us who took sex education in high school know, those topics about pleasuring our partner certainly weren't covered in those bumbling and pathetic attempts to teach sex and birth control 101 responsibly to high school kids whose hormones were running rampant. And those of us whose parents tried, however awkwardly, to educate us in sexuality recall those sessions to be mainly fear-based "don't get pregnant or don't impregnate anyone or catch any of those horrible diseases" and often lame exhortations to remain pure as the proverbial driven snow until marriage. Right? Perhaps somewhere between an estimated 1–5 percent of us had really cool parents back then who understood that it made sense to pass along healthy and useful information about sex and reliable birth control. That's my statistical guess. I could be wrong. But I think I'm right, at least, for those who grew up when I did, from the late 1940s through the 1960s.

Some of Us Are Just Too Serious, It's Time to Come Out and Play

Many of us are so busy being adults, going about our daily lives, noses to the grindstone, putting food on the table, doing errands, paying our bills, and having a little fun occasionally. Many of us have kids. Free time is spent on exercise, sports, hobbies or watching/ attending sporting events, or dining and drinking at the local watering spot.

Often there just doesn't seem to be room for sexual expression. Or making it a priority seems frivolous and silly. Far from it. Sexual expression is essential to your well-being, and squashing it as if it didn't need to exist frequently results in overcompensating, often compulsively, in some other area of your life. Instead of having great sex, many of us exercise compulsively, drink, smoke, or overeat; some of us even clean our houses to a point that we could eat off our floors, but somehow we just can't find the time or space for a great sex life. It's time to rethink that entire scenario and reorganize our priorities.

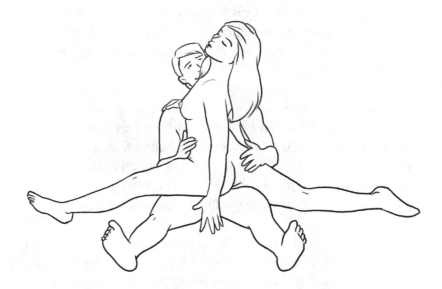

Rule 4: Plan sex *play* for at least two hours a week—both singles and couples.

If you aren't ready to commit, at the very least, two hours a week to your sex life, you might as well put this book down right now. I already talked about wham bam, thank you, ma'am, being a poor excuse for a sex life, even though so many people settle for just that, mainly to get it over with, before turning over to go to sleep. If your married sex life is limited to dull sex on Valentine's Day, your birthday and your anniversary, rare occurrences when the kids are away, you are missing out on literally scores of opportunities for healthy sex play. This means you are losing endless chances to be closer to your partner, not only physically but also emotionally. Healthy sex play actually builds relationships.

Another important item: If your single sex life doesn't include some serious and regular *masturbation* sessions, you are missing out on a release that is healthy and essential to your well-being. Orgasms not only lower blood pressure, they also release endorphins, letting you drift to a peaceful sleep afterward. Masturbation also relieves menstrual discomfort.[1, 2]

The approach to one's sex life as something to just do quickly and get over with is not only uninspired, it is downright unhealthy. And to have no sex life is a total abomination (I hope that one day, I won't be sorry I said that). According to WebMD Daily, "What Happens When You Stop Having Sex," there are a number of seriously negative outcomes that can result when you stop having sex, from a weakened immune system, increased blood pressure, heart disease, to a compromised *prostate gland*. Mental issues, including memory loss and anxiety, can also result. Sex isn't something to be ashamed of, embarrassed about, or ignored away. An exciting sex life,

---

[1] Cramps, bloating and more; important sexual and other information.
[2] https://www.independent.co.uk/life-style/love-sex/the-health-benefits-of-masturbation-a7050761.html.

at any age of adulthood, is essential to reaching your peak of physical and emotional health. Great sex is a fundamental human need. But so many of us are giant prudes.

Assignment 2: Find time to treat yourself and masturbate at least once a week. Dress up in sexy clothes and use your full-length mirror to get turned on (a form of autoeroticism/dressing up adds tremendously to the entire experience).
An added bonus: Take photographs of your images.

CHAPTER 9
A GOOD SEXUAL PARTNER IS DIFFICULT TO FIND

If you don't already have one, a good sexual partner is amazingly difficult to find. Ask anyone you know. This is true when you are looking for a hot sexual encounter. It's especially true when you are looking for a long-term relationship or partner in marriage. Bad sex, or *sexual incompatibility*, is blamed for the end of both short-term and long-term relationships.

Unhappy marriages are often virtually sexless and a truly miserable existence that forms the breeding ground for *extramarital affairs*. But with all of that said, what does it take to be a good sexual partner? Actually that question is quite easy to answer, which means we will get to the main point of this book immediately.

Oral Sex Worth Writing Home About

Ask a woman if she ever had a partner who was a completely comfortable and unselfish lover. The key questions to ask are: "Did he go down on you and perform *oral sex* and like or even love doing it? Did he do it with the gusto of a hound dog? Did he eat you like you were a banquet?" If she had such a partner, the smile on her face will speak volumes. Or perhaps she is reticent to give up these details. The more she appears to be a Cheshire cat, trying to hide the truth, the more you know that she has had great oral sex and doesn't want to share with you about it in details.

Rule 5: Men with a small or even an average penis can make up for it with great oral techniques.

Ask a man if he ever had a partner who was a completely comfortable and unselfish lover. The key questions to ask are: "Did she suck your cock and perform oral sex and like, or even better, love, doing it? Did she *deep-throat* your *cock* and gently suck your *balls*? Did she look at you while sucking you with a look of horny desire on her face?" If he did have such a partner, the smile on his face will speak volumes.

I can predict what many of you are thinking—explosions! Fireworks! Ecstasy! Or shock and awe! Revulsion! Disgust! Or perhaps a bit of both, or probably somewhere in between the two in a no-man's-land of *prudery* and sexual ignorance, or perhaps these details elicit pangs of jealousy?

Let's face facts: People's reactions to the idea of great oral sex are all over the map. Men with a smaller penis definitely need to develop their oral skills since confident women invariably love it when their man goes down on them. And if she says she doesn't feel those things about it, then I venture to say that there isn't a man alive that doesn't like his cock sucked. If he says he doesn't, he's probably lying or never had it done right.

In fact, a man's performance of oral sex can almost make or break a relationship. A man who doesn't do it is seriously cheating his woman out of a huge experience of sexual satisfaction. And a woman who turns her nose up and refuses to suck her guy's penis is—and I'm sorry that I have to say this—just plain stupid. Every man loves his cock to be the center of the universe. He will love you for it, so just do it.

Since oral sex is one of the most important—and in my opinion—the principal key to successful sexual expression and, therefore, at the core *raison d'*être of this book, we will go into it extensively on pages 67 through 275.

Back to reality. But before we segue into another topic, let's explore quickly the population of people who simply don't like to perform oral sex. I will venture to say that they are either not doing it right or need some serious education in order to *suck cock* and/or *eat pussy* correctly. Or their past experiences have been disastrous at best because it seemed disgusting or degrading. That said, it's sort of like eating an oyster. Some people really love raw oysters and the entire process of eating them, and other people don't even like the thought of it. So I say that some serious relearning is in order.

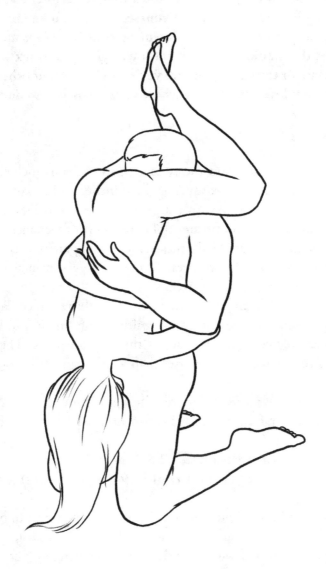

Men! Women! Learn how to give oral sex: This is the key to the main message of this book. If you know you like receiving oral sex, it only follows that it's time to reconcile yourself to learning how to love doing it yourself, if only to be able to pleasure your partner. After all, pleasuring your partner is most of the title of this book. There is great joy in giving oral sex when you are aware of the sheer pleasure you're giving to that other person whom you love. Besides the whole scenario is just so damn hot.

Penis Size

We've all heard how the average penis size is six inches, and the variations range from as small as three inches and as large as, well, nearly a foot long. Men with a large penis love to show it off as much as possible. And men who are confident show off a smaller penis as if it were larger. It might be the masculine idea of potent force that men are so focused on their penises. That organ gives immense pleasure and is a life force creator as well.

The reader may wish to visit the website called Penis Size Comparison: Size Me Up[1] for a wealth of information to help you get over preconceived ideas about the magical penis. The average penis size is considerably shorter than we thought. It is <u>not</u> <u>even</u> six inches.

Medical News Today and the National Center for Biotechnology Information (NCBI)[2] also have pertinent details about size averages:

- An average penis size of 8.8 cm (3.5 inches) when *flaccid*
- **An average penis size of 12.9 cm (5.1 inches) when *erect***

I don't know about you, but I find those numbers to be inconceivable. How do you feel about it? This gives a pass to you guys who parade around with your six-inch cocks hanging out. Now we understand your pride.

---

[1] www.sizemeup.info.
[2] https://pubmed.ncbi.nlm.nih.gov/8709382/.

How to Measure Your Penis

The medically correct method of measuring your penis is to place a ruler firmly against the pubic bone on the top side of the erect penis, and measure to the tip of the head. Measuring from underneath is not the correct way. You may wish to do this with your penis when it is both flaccid and erect. No stretching allowed.

Challenge 1: Gentlemen, measure your penis, both flaccid and erect.

CHAPTER 10
GAINING EXPERIENCE WITH CUB-COUGAR RELATIONSHIPS

What are some ways to gain experience? For young men, perhaps a willing older woman; a cougar teaching her cub is a great solution to learning the ropes of sex. Interestingly, while the opposite phenomenon isn't considered proper, cougar/cub doesn't seem to be seriously frowned upon in our society. In the cougar-cub world, a cub approaches the older woman and initiates the relationship because he finds that an older woman is more desirable, confident, comfortable, and safe than a peer/similar-age relationship. One big impetus to such a relationship is that there's no fear of pregnancy or monthly periods to deal with. If the cougar is a grandmother living apart from her grandchildren, another benefit is that children are unlikely additions to the mix to distract them from the pleasure they are giving to each other.

Figuring Out the Scene

Making a decision to become a cougar is a big one. It requires an entirely new mindset of what's attractive, what's appropriate, and what's sexy. It requires that you determine what age group interests you. If you are a hot sixty-five-year-old, you may wish to meet men in their forties and fifties, instead of twenties and thirties, because the older ones, with all their maturity, also have valuable experience. Initially, though, you may wish to experience a couple of eager younger ones for the pure fun of it. There are no rules. Only suggestions.

There's a website that is rich in useful information. It is called "16 Reasons Young Men are Attracted to Older Women"[1] I won't blame you if you get lost here for a while.

16 Reasons Young Men Are Attracted to Older Women

1. He loves your experience
2. You know what he wants (because you want it too)
3. He can learn a lot
4. You both know what you want
5. He respects you for all that you've achieved
6. He learns a new perspective
7. You are confident and independent
8. You are more emotionally mature
9. You have refined tastes
10. You can have intellectual discussions
11. You are financially stable
12. They don't have to worry about having children
13. They love your emotional support
14. You're good at cooking
15. She's more direct and knows what she wants
16. You both envision a future of possibility

Additional qualities of accomplished cougars recently noted by an experienced cub:

- Confident
- Comfortable in her own skin

---

[1] https://hackspirit.com/cougar-love-young-men-older-successful-women-perfect-dating-combination/.

- Motivated
- Curious about life
- Passionate
- Person of substance
- Smart
- Great sense of humor
- Open-minded

> I have always preferred older women, ever since I was in my teens. Older women are way more interesting intellectually and other ways. They know what they want and don't want. And aren't afraid to say it or go get it. I love that. They don't play games, and they are much more sensual and sexual. It's what most men don't understand. I find women in their seventies are less inhibited than those in their twenties and thirties and more in touch with their bodies. (Anonymous cub, forty-four years old)

I'd like to add the fact that being a cub is the lifestyle of men of various age ranges, and these men have seldom been married or had kids. They have known what they want from an early age. And they are so turned on by an older woman who is a sexy cougar. It's an increasingly common sexual preference. I think it's absolutely fascinating.

The age spread between two partners in a cougar-cub relationship actually ranges from around ten to thirty years or more. Yes, this is a real and thriving phenomenon. There's a special section in this book that goes into this in more detail (see pages xx and xxx).

Thoughts from a Seventy-Year-Old Woman about Oral Sex

The older I get, the more I love oral sex, both giving and receiving it. The first time it happened to me, when I was an adolescent,

I was overwhelmed with embarrassment. I mean, my pussy seemed like a rank open wound in my body. I couldn't get over how disgusting I thought it was and how could I expect that someone else might like to lick and kiss me down there? But then I matured sexually and learned what an almost-endless instrument of pleasure that my body is. I finally understood that all I needed to do was wash myself properly before sex. Maybe as long as thirty minutes of masturbation, oral sex, and fucking—explosion. And, boy oh boy, does that feel good. I want more of that.

CHAPTER 11
SEXUAL PREFERENCES

Now for the Nuts and Bolts of Essential Basic Sexual Knowledge

The Human Rights Campaign defines sexual orientation as "an inherent or immutable enduring emotional, romantic or sexual attraction to another specific group of people."

Most of us are born into and grow up with our own sexual orientation or preference clearly identified. But this is not always the case, and the road to sexual maturity can be quite bumpy at times. According to an article on sexual orientation on Planned Parenthood's website, "Sexual orientation is about who you're attracted to and want to have relationships with." That sounds amazingly simple, doesn't it?

What Does It Mean to Be Straight/Heterosexual?

Most heterosexuals know, from an early age, that they are either masculine or feminine based on their *genitals* and on the *hormones* that begin to course through their bodies, as early as seven years old in girls and nine years old in boys.[1] Not only does heterosexuality as a sexual orientation refer to a person's emotional, romantic, and

---

[1] "Everything You Wanted to Know About Puberty (for Teens)," KidsHealth.

sexual attractions to persons of the opposite sex, it also refers to a person's sense of identity, related behaviors, and membership in a community of others who share those attractions.[2] When you think about it, it seems that heterosexuals have it really easy compared to all of the other sexual orientations. Everything throughout society supports and reinforces the heterosexual archetype.

Early Experiences

For example, it is common and, therefore, perfectly normal during early sexual development to have same-sex exploratory experiences. These experiences are not regarded as homosexual in nature. In a Swedish study described in an online article entitled "Sexual experiences in childhood: young adults' recollections," Svedin Larsson found that nearly 83 percent of young people reported early mutual experiences with a same-age friend. Girls generally had more same-sex experiences than boys did. Larsson's study validated the idea that generally, "the years before puberty seem to be years of frequent mutual sexual exploration and experimentation."[3]

> I remember the girl that I had my two childhood (sexual) exploration sessions with when we were about ten years old. Amazingly she and I are still in touch today, a whopping sixty-three years later (the author).

Unfortunately Larsson also found an increase of *childhood sexually abusive experiences*; a small percentage (8.2 percent) of children is forced to participate in sexual activities. In fact:

> Some kind of coercive sexual experiences appears to be part of growing up for quite a few children. According to Developmental-Behavioral Pediatrics, 2008, "*sexual play* is dis-

---

[2] "Heterosexuality," Wikipedia.
[3] ncbi.nlm.nig.gov.

tinguished from problematic behaviors in that childhood sexual play involves behaviors that occur spontaneously and intermittently, are mutual and noncoercive when they involve other children, and do not cause emotional distress.[4]

Sexual Urges of Children

During *puberty*, the body starts to produce more sex hormones, and one of the results can be a greater interest in and curiosity about sexuality. *Masturbation* is a regular activity of most boys who, once they discover what orgasm is like, find it difficult to keep the activity down to a dull roar.

Unfortunately sites such as Pornhub[5] are especially useful for young people (over eighteen) wishing to explore their sexual urges.

An online article from HealthyChildren.org acknowledges how "at a very young age, children begin to explore their bodies by touching, poking, pulling, and rubbing their body parts, including their genitals."[6] Apparently pediatricians say that all kinds of behavior around genitals is common in two through six-year-olds.[7] Surprise! If a parent doesn't jump nervously to correct such behavior, it seems perfectly natural if you think about it. Usually it's best to suggest gently to the child that that activity belongs in private. But no guilt, shaming, or punishment, parents, please.

---

[4] https://www.sciencedirect.com/topics/psychology/sexual-play.

[5] "The world's leading free porn site is not for children."

[6] "Sexual Behaviors in Young Children: What's Normal, What's Not?"

[7] https://www.healthychildren.org/English/ages-stages/preschool/Pages/Sexual-Behaviors-Young-Children.aspx.

What Does It Mean to Be Gay/Homosexual?

A significant percentage of the population is *gay (homosexual)*. That said, the question quickly becomes: what percentage are we talking about? The answer to this, it turns out, depends on who is making the claims. According to a 1993 *Janus Report*, 9 percent of males and 5 percent of females identify as gay, having at least occasional gay sexual relationships.[8]

But Alfred Kinsey, the famous sex researcher, claimed 10 percent of the male population is gay in his groundbreaking 1948 book entitled *Sexual Behavior in the Human Male*. The US Census Bureau found in 2000 that homosexual couples constitute less than 1 percent of American households. And the Family Research Report claimed in 2002 that around 2–3 percent of men and 2 percent of women are homosexual or bisexual.

In Broward County, Florida, where the city of Wilton Manors has become the residential favorite of thousands of gay people, it certainly seems that those statistics are way, way off. Known as a gay village, and second in the US for its percentage of gay couples as a proportion of total population, with 140 gay couples per 1,000 residents, a full 14 percent of the nearly 13,000 inhabitants. Nearby the city of Fort Lauderdale elected its first gay mayor in 2018, and reelected him; so evidently, the entire area is gay friendly, which is a very happy state of affairs for LGBTQ people.

Finally the National Gay and Lesbian Task Force estimated in 2002 that between 3 percent and 8 percent of both sexes in the total population is gay or bisexual.[9] But apparently, when Gallup, the famous polling company, asked Americans for their best estimate of the American gay and lesbian population in 2002, the results made all the figures mentioned above look conservative. The claim was that one in five people, or 25 percent of men and women are homosexual. Can you imagine what it must be like to remain closeted well after

---

[8] Jennifer Robison, "What Percentage of the Population is Gay?" News.gallup. com.

[9] Ibid.

coming out as gay to a very limited group of people? Being gay brings numerous issues with it, and some of these are discussed here.

> **For the most complete list of terms that people call themselves or others, visit this link. See below.**[10]

There are other ways of personal stories about self-discovery, including the concept that fairly often, a person who begins life straight culminates with being gay. For example, there are many gay adults who initially committed to a conventional heterosexual married relationship, many of them having children, only to, sometime later, come out of the closet and, after the end of the marriage, either adopt a solo gay sex life or have homosexual relationships. And since gay marriage is now legal in a growing number of states, that population is increasing by leaps and bounds. People who lived together "in sin" are finally legally cleared to marry and enjoy all that marriage brings.

What is euphemistically called the *gay lifestyle* has changed in the age of AIDS. Gay bathhouses, nightclubs, and tea dances have always been gathering places for gay men to meet and carouse. But nowadays, gay men are much more apt to practice safe sex with prescription medication and condoms, especially if they are carriers of HIV, which is no longer the kind of death sentence that it once was. To guard against contracting HIV, increasing numbers of gay men are settling down in monogamous relationships instead of adopting a promiscuous sex life.

> **According to an online article by therapist Tom Bruett, those wishing to make their sexual encounters safer, may decide to take a daily pill called PrEP, or pre-exposure prophylaxis, a treatment to prevent HIV infection that was**

---

[10] https://www.umass.edu/stonewall/sites/default/files/documents/allyship_term_handout.pdf.

> **approved by the *FDA* in 2014 (condom use to prevent STIs or STDs is also seriously recommended).**[11]

In Bruett's article, "Understanding the monogamy spectrum in gay relationships and deciding what's best for you," three gay life-styles are identified: Monogamy—a committed relationship with one person. Monogamish—couples who are mostly monogamous. Ethical nonmonogamy—a relationship that is fair, open, and transparent, with no intentions to hurt the other person.

The Couples Study,[12] a website compiled by Blake Spears and Lanz Lowen, found that younger gay men are increasingly seeking and having more monogamous relationships than their elders. "Gay marriage is becoming the norm." They conclude that "both gay monogamous and non-monogamous relationships have the potential for long-term success."[13]

That study found that "47% reported open relationships, 45% were monogamous, and the remaining 8% were unsure what type relationships they were in."

> ***Homophobia* is the "irrational hatred, intolerance, and fear" of lesbian, gay, bisexual and transgender (LGBT) people, and is a form of discrimination.**[14]

---

[11] www.tombruetttherapy.com.

[12] A treasure trove of information about being gay or lesbian.

[13] Site URL is thecouplesstudy.com.

[14] Avert.org.

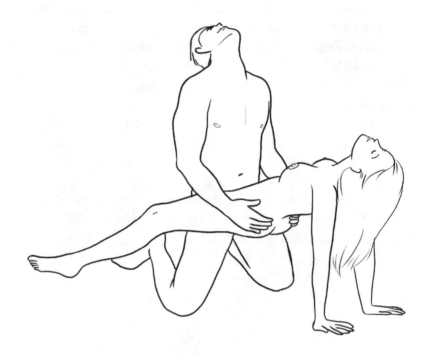

In the Couples Study, Bruett offers a complete guide to feeling safe in relationships that includes ground rules, communication, honesty, and acknowledgement of jealousy. Sounds worthwhile, doesn't it?

In the appendix there is an article entitled "The Gay Paradox," by an anonymous contributor, a sixty-four-year-old active gay man, who is about to retire. He lives near Wilton Manors, Florida.

What Does It Mean to Be Bisexual?

The best answer to this question varies, depending upon who is asking and who is answering it. The Bisexual Resource Center (www.biresource.org) actually goes to extremes to try to explain and demystify this subject.

> When talking about *bisexuality*, it is sometimes useful to distinguish between behavior, attraction, and identity. Someone who has had sexual experience with or even just attractions to people of more than one gender can be described as bisexual+, but may not identify that way. Likewise, one can identify as bisexual+ regardless of sexual experience. Furthermore, identities can change over time or be used in different contexts, whether personal, community, or political. Definitions can change too.

Clearly bisexuality cannot be defined easily or simply.

"Some identify as bisexual, while others use *pansexual, queer, fluid,* or no label at all to describe their attractions to more than one gender." Attractions can include masculinity and femininity, or *androgyny* or the blending of genders, or even biological sex. To explain, sex is between your legs; gender is between your ears. Sex and gender don't always correspond.[15] Please visit the www.biresource.org

---

[15] https://biresource.org/resources/youth/what-is-bisexuality/.

website to understand all the complicated permutations of bisexuality since it claims that "dictionary definitions of bisexuality that rely on an idea of 'both sexes'" are inadequate. The point is that romantic and/or sexual attraction varies in time, manner, and degree.[16]

On the Bisexual Resource Center blog, there's an article entitled "Coming Out as a Bisexual Man: The 5 Reasons Why We Don't," by Mark Lees, MA, that points out that according to a Pew Research Center Survey, bisexual men are the least of the LGBTQ community to be *out* to (even) those closest to them, despite the fact that it is the largest sector of the community. Apparently only 28 percent of bisexual people and 12 percent of bisexual men tell their friends, family, and coworkers.[17] Please visit this site to learn more about coming out as a bisexual man.

The Wikipedia analysis of demographics of sexual orientation is much simpler in its analysis, stating that "bisexuals accounted for 1.3% of the male population and 2.2% of the female population, but reinforces the assertion that men reported less while women reported more about their same-sex experience and same-sex attraction."[18]

What Does It Mean to Be Transgender?

Sexual orientation is different from *gender* and *gender identity*.[19] This is particularly the case with *transgender* individuals. A transgender person is faced with the strong feeling that they were born into the wrong body, often at a very young age. As increasing numbers indicate, the parents of transgender children are taking their children's assertions seriously and helping them, with specialized medical help, to realize their desires to transition into the opposite sex. Whether this ultimately includes gender reassignment surgery or not, it often includes hormone blockers and treatment to stop *menstruation* in the

---

[16] Ibid.

[17] https://biresource.org/coming-out-as-a-bisexual-man-the-5-reasons-why-we-dont/.

[18] https://en.wikipedia.org/wiki/Demographics_of_sexual_orientation.

[19] "Sexual Orientation," Planned Parenthood.

female body and hormone blockers to stop sexual development in the male body, including such features as a beard, Adam's apple, and well-developed male genitals.

The principal reason to begin in childhood is hormonal. Some hormones are blocked and others added to achieve the desired result as the child grows up. Waiting until one is already passed or passing puberty creates additional problems later on.

Of course, there are many transgender individuals who make their transition in adulthood. But this is not the ideal way in which to accomplish transition because the human body's main sexual development takes place during puberty, "the period during which adolescents reach sexual maturity and become capable of reproduction."[20]

Famed Olympic athlete Bruce Jenner, now Caitlyn Marie Jenner, came out as a transwoman in 2015, saying that she had dealt with lifelong *gender dysphoria*, the distress suffered due to the mismatch between gender identity and the sex assigned at birth.[21] Jenner underwent cosmetic surgery and *sex reassignment surgery* in 2017, and despite becoming a transwoman, he isn't sexually attracted to men.[22]

Popular TV personality known as Jazz Jennings (Jennings is a pseudonym), born October 6, 2000, and the youngest publicly documented transgendered individual, has had details of her transition televised on the Learning Channel, endearing herself to a large audience who have watched in fascination as this young woman has been enthusiastically and financially supported by her parents in her decision to be a girl, despite being born a boy. In the process, she has become a YouTube personality, spokesmodel, and LGBT rights activist.[23]

She cowrote a book entitled *Jazz: My Life as a (Transgender) Teen*. Her TV show, entitled *I Am Jazz*, has achieved widespread public understanding of what it is like to be a transgender male going

---

[20] *Oxford Dictionary.*
[21] https://www.nhs.uk/conditions/gender-dysphoria/.
[22] https://en.wikipedia.org/wiki/Caitlyn_Jenner#Coming_out_as_a_transgender_woman.
[23] https://en.wikipedia.org/wiki/Jazz_Jennings.

through both top and bottom surgery to become a female with breasts and a sexually functioning vagina (note: it should be clear that this surgery does not confer the ability to become pregnant or any other female sexual functions).

According to the *Human Rights Campaign*, "being transgender does not imply any specific sexual orientation. Therefore, transgender people may identify as straight, gay, lesbian, bisexual, etc." (sexual orientation and gender identity definitions, hrc.org [note: in addition, the hrc.org site offers an impressive glossary of terms and a Coming Out Center for information on living openly and authentically).

What Does It Mean to Be Pansexual?

"*Pansexuality*, or *omnisexuality*, is the sexual, romantic or emotional attraction towards people regardless of their sex or gender identity. Pansexual people may refer to themselves as gender-blind, asserting that gender and sex are not determining factors in their romantic or sexual attraction to others."[24] Pansexuality removes limitations in sexual choice.[25] Their attraction to another person is based on personality, not gender.

According to Wikipedia, "pansexuality may be considered a sexual orientation in its own right or a branch of bisexuality, to indicate an alternative sexual identity." Pansexual people reject what's known as the *gender binary*, which is "the classification of gender into two distinct, opposite, and disconnected forms of masculine and feminine, whether by social system or cultural belief."

Identifying as pansexual, Jazz Jennings has had attractions to males and females and had her first boyfriend documented on the TV show. It was problematic because the young man's mother insisted that Jazz actually had to be a "gay male" as a transgender male to

---

[24] https://en.wikipedia.org/wiki/Pansexuality.
[25] *Oxford*.

female. According to the *National Center for Transgender Equality*, 25 percent of American transgender people identify as bisexual.[26]

What Does It Mean to Be Polyamorous?

According to Wikipedia, "*polyamory* is the practice of, or desire for, interpersonal relationships that involve physical and/or emotional intimacy with more than one partner, with the consent to engage in sexual activity of all partners involved." The most recognizable description for polyamory is an *open relationship*, which, by definition, rejects the view that sexual and relational exclusivity are necessary for deep, committed, long-term loving relationships.[27]

Polyamory is an umbrella term for *nonmonogamous, multipartner relationships, or nonexclusive* sexual or romantic relationships. Apparently few studies have been conducted on the prevalence of open polyamory because it is relatively rare, while a study in Finland in 1992 found that 8.9 percent of those studied agreed with the statement "I could maintain several sexual relationships at the same time."

Interestingly, "polyamory offers release from the monogamist expectation that one person must meet all of an individual's needs (sex, emotional support, primary friendship, intellectual stimulation, companionship, social presentation)."[28]

Realizing that no one person can meet all of these needs, these most enlightened polyamorous people negotiate with their partners to eliminate jealousy, insecurity, and possessiveness and have it all. Is humanity ready for such a relationship? Is it too unconventional to become commonplace? Only time will reveal the answer to that question.

How do you feel about polyamory? Is it appealing to you because you believe that most people (principally men) practice polyamory without admitting it to their spouse. Why is it that a man who is

---

[26] https://thetaskforceblog.org/2013/06/05/wonky-wednesday-trans-people-sexual-orientation/.

[27] https://en.wikipedia.org/wiki/Polyamory.

[28] https://en.wikipedia.org/wiki/Polyamory#Prevalence.

dating a variety of women is acceptable while a woman who behaves that way is said to be a slut? Just asking.

What about Nonbinary or Genderqueer?

According to online research, the terms *nonbinary* and *genderqueer* are interchangeable. They represent a "spectrum of gender identities that are not exclusively masculine or feminine" and, therefore, outside of the gender binary. They can fall under the transgender umbrella, since many nonbinary people identified with a gender that is different from their assigned sex" (dear readers, I must confess that most of this is Greek to me, and I hope you will forgive me for bringing it up in the first place. Hopefully a population of nonbinary or genderqueer readers will emerge and straighten me out. Signed, P. H. Fisk, author).

CHAPTER 12
SEX HORMONES

Let's discuss sex hormones, their functions, and why they are so important to the sexual and physical functioning of every human being. Hormones are chemical substances—chemical messengers—secreted by one tissue and travelling in bodily fluids to affect another tissue in the body. Many hormones are significant to both men and women, especially those hormones affecting growth and behavior. Because they are secreted in short bursts, or pulses, that vary from minute to minute, amounts and levels of hormones are continually changing. Hormone release varies between night and day and stages of a woman's *menstrual cycle.*[1]

Produced by a group of *glands* also known as the *endocrine system*, hormones course through your bloodstream and turn on switches to the genetic machinery that regulate everything from reproduction to emotions, general health, and well-being. They may be thought of as the life-giving force that animates you physically, mentally, and emotionally.[2]

---

[1] https://www.webmd.com/women/guide/normal-testosterone-and-estrogen-levels-in-women#1-2.

[2] "Is Pellet Hormone Therapy for Me? What You Should Know About Bioequivalent Hormones" (patient brochure).

As hormone production decreases, the body often begins to slow down its rejuvenation and repair of tissues and organs. This can cause health to decline and aging to accelerate.

Menopause is that dreaded change of life that has potential to rob a woman of her sexual desire. Some common effects of low hormones during menopause include hot flashes, night sweats, loss of interest in sex, pain during sex, problems sleeping, loss of energy, fatigue, loss of muscle mass, weight gain, foggy thinking, mood changes, and memory loss.[3]

Estrogen

Estrogen is the primary female hormone, promoting the growth and health of the female reproductive organs and keeps the vagina moisturized, elastic (stretchy), and well supplied with blood.[4]

Estrogen is an entire class of related hormones that includes estriol, estradiol, and estrone. Estradiol is made from the (human) placenta produced during pregnancy. Estradiol is the primary sex hormone of childbearing women, formed from developing ovarian follicles. Estradiol is responsible for female characteristics and sexual functioning. It is also important to women's bone health. Unfortunately it also contributes to most gynecologic problems, including endometriosis and fibroids and even female cancers. Estrone is widespread throughout the body. It is the main estrogen that remains present after menopause.[5]

Estrogen:

- Is responsible for the sexual development of girls during puberty.
- Controls the growth of the uterine lining during the menstrual cycle and at the beginning of a pregnancy.

---

[3] https://my.clevelandclinic.org/health/articles/15660-bioidentical-hormones.
[4] http://www.menopause.org/for-women/sexual-health-menopause-online/changes-at-midlife/changes-in-hormone-levels.
[5] https://www.webmd.com/women/guide/normal-testosterone-and-estrogen-levels-in-women#1-3.

- Causes breast changes in pregnant teenagers and women.
- Is involved in bone and cholesterol metabolism working in conjunction with calcium, vitamin D, and other minerals to keep bones strong.
- Regulates food intake, body weight, glucose metabolism, and insulin sensitivity.[6]

There are various reasons why *estrogen levels* fall. Pregnancy failure, extreme exercising, perimenopause,[7] and menopause are some of them. Women experience low levels of estrogen after childbirth and during breastfeeding.[8] This is nature's way of encouraging mothers to focus on caring for their newborns instead of sex.

Other common symptoms of low estrogen include painful sex due to lack of vaginal lubrication, increased urinary tract infections (also called UTIs), irregular or absent menstrual periods, breast tenderness, headaches, accentuation of preexisting *migraines, depression,* trouble concentrating, and fatigue. It can also lead to *infertility* in women if left untreated.[9]

Estrogen rises during puberty during breast development and other maturing features as well as in women who are extremely overweight, have certain tumors, or are pregnant. Certain drugs can cause increased estrogen levels as well.[10]

In addition to testosterone, which I will discuss next, men produce estrogen, which works with the testosterone to develop a man's body for sexual growth and development. [11]

---

[6] https://www.healthline.com/health/womens-health/low-estrogen-symptoms.

[7] Perimenopause begins several years before menopause when ovaries begin to make less estrogen.

[8] https://www.webmd.com/women/guide/normal-testosterone-and-estrogen-levels-in-women#1-4.

[9] https://www.healthline.com/health/womens-health/low-estrogen-symptoms# causes.

[10] https://www.webmd.com/women/guide/normal-testosterone-and-estrogen-levels-in-women#2-7.

[11] Wikipedia.

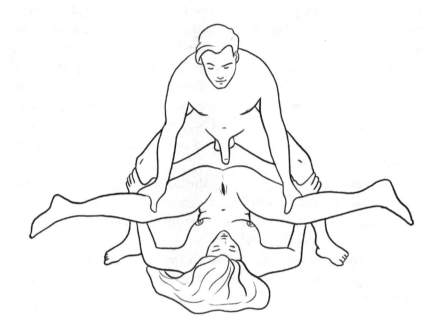

Testosterone

> *Testosterone* is a naturally occurring sex hormone that is produced in a man's testicles. Small amounts of testosterone are also produced in a woman's ovaries and adrenal system.[12]

According to Wikipedia, testosterone is the primary male sex hormone[13] responsible for developing male reproductive organs, such as the testes and the prostate,[14] and as an *anabolic steroid*,[15] it increases protein within cells and promotes secondary sexual characteristics, such as increased muscle and bone mass and body hair. As such, it also stimulates linear growth and bone maturation. Its androgenic effects include maturation of the sex organs (the penis and *scrotum*) during fetal development and during puberty, when the voice deepens, facial and underarm hair grows.

Testosterone is also involved in health and well-being and the prevention of the loss of bone mass called osteoporosis.[16] Osteoporosis increases after menopause[17] because of lower levels of estrogen.

In women, age-related (not menopause-related) declines in testosterone may dampen *libido*, or sex drive, although this remains controversial.[18]

Testosterone has very complex roles to play from fetal development, into early infancy, before and during puberty, and throughout adulthood. Some of the familiar roles that it plays include the development of spermatogenic tissue in testicles, male fertility, penis or clitoris enlargement, increased libido, and frequency of erection or clitoral engorgement (i.e., sexual arousal).

---

[12] https://www.drugs.com/testosterone.html.

[13] https://en.wikipedia.org/wiki/Testosterone.

[14] https://en.wikipedia.org/wiki/Male.

[15] https://en.wikipedia.org/wiki/Anabolic_steroid.

[16] https://en.wikipedia.org/wiki/Osteoporosis.

[17] https://en.wikipedia.org/wiki/Menopause.

[18] http://www.menopause.org/for-women/sexual-health-menopause-online/changes-at-midlife/changes-in-hormone-levels.

This is where testosterone especially counts in our discussions of sexuality. Higher levels of testosterone in men are associated with periods of sexual activity. And the androgens made available in testosterone "may" modulate the physiology of vaginal tissue and contribute to genital sexual arousal.[19]

Progesterone

> *Progesterone* is a hormone released by the ovaries. Changing progesterone levels can contribute to abnormal menstrual periods and menopausal symptoms. Progesterone is also necessary for implantation of the fertilized egg in the uterus and for maintaining pregnancy.[20]

According to an Internet newsletter posted by *Medical News Today*, "Progesterone is the main pro-gestational steroid hormone secreted by the female reproductive system. It is linked to the menstrual cycle, pregnancy, and development of an embryo… The ovaries, placenta, and adrenal glands produce progesterone to regulate the condition of the endometrium, which is the inner lining of the uterus."[21]

The presence or absence of progesterone determines the presence or absence of blood in the walls of the uterus and allows for the implantation of an egg in the wall of the uterus. It also prevents other eggs from maturing after pregnancy occurs and prepares the breast tissue for lactation. Progesterone levels drop just before menopause, causing menopausal symptoms, including hot flashes and night sweats.[22]

---

[19] https://en.wikipedia.org/wiki/Testosterone.
[20] https://www.webmd.com/vitamins/ai/ingredientmono-760/progesterone.
[21] https://www.medicalnewstoday.com/articles/277737.php.
[22] https://www.medicalnewstoday.com/articles/277737.php#what_is_progesterone.

CHAPTER 13
FEMALE ANATOMY
AND FUNCTIONS

Breasts

Both females and males develop breasts from the same embryological tissues. In females, breasts serve as the mammary gland, which produces and secretes milk to feed infants. Breasts develop during puberty with the help of estrogen and growth hormone.[1]

> Along with their major function in providing nutrition for infants, female breasts have social and sexual characteristics...and can figure prominently in the perception of a woman's body and her sexual attractiveness.[2]

Sexual attractiveness or sex appeal is an individual's ability to attract the sexual or *erotic* interests of other people and is a factor in sexual selection or mate choice. Sexual

---

[1] https://en.wikipedia.org/wiki/Breast.
[2] Ibid.

attraction is based on sexual desire or the quality of arousing such interest.[3]

We have all heard about men's different preferences for different body parts. Some men identify as a breast man, while others are ass men, and still others respond to a woman's legs or other body parts. Much of this is highly charged with vivid sex talk to increase excitement levels.

Nipples

Aside from being the organ that feeds milk to infants, nipples are a major *erogenous zone*. Surrounded by the areola, nipples actually provide both males and females sexual arousal through stimulation.[4] A study of over three hundred men and women (seventeen to twenty-nine) found that nipple stimulation enhanced sexual arousal in 82 percent of women and 52 percent of men. Seven to 8 percent said it decreased arousal.[5] This is due to the heightened sensitivity of the nipple when stimulated.

Your nipples can be flat, protruding, inverted, or unclassified (multiple or divided)…one breast with a protruding nipple and the other with an inverted, making the total combination of nipple types up to eight.[6]

Pussy

Now let's get down to the real nitty-gritty. The word *pussy* is used to describe both the entire female sexual organ and parts outside where hair grows. Other common names for the sex organ include box, twat, snatch, cunt, and slice of heaven.[7] It is also commonly

---

[3] https://en.wikipedia.org/wiki/Sexual_attraction.

[4] https://en.wikipedia.org/wiki/Nipple.

[5] https://www.healthline.com/health/nipple-facts-male-and-female#9.

[6] https://www.healthline.com/health/nipple-facts-male-and-female#2.

[7] https://www.urbandictionary.com/define.php?term=Pussy.

and incorrectly called a *vagina* because the vagina is the birth canal and the area where the male penis enters the female during intercourse. That leaves an entire outer and inner part of the female sexual organs.

Joke: The "pussy is something that (male) babies spend 9 months getting out of, and the rest of their lives trying to get back into" (source unknown).

Vulva

The *vulva* is the external part of the female *genitalia*. It protects a woman's sexual organs, urinary opening, vestibule and vagina and is the center of much of a woman's sexual response. The outer and inner 'lips' of the vulva are called the labia majora and labia minora. The vestibule surrounds the opening of the vagina, or introitus, and the opening of the urethra, or urethral meatus. The perineum is the area extending from beneath the vulva to the anus.[8]

It's important to know that women's vulvas vary tremendously due to variations in the appearance of the lips of the vulva. Some women's labia majora and minora are almost nonexistent, others are quite abbreviated; while still others are downright floppy and actually hang down.

While many women (and their men) prefer the natural hairy look for the vulva, in recent years, women have increasingly opted to shave their pubic hair, giving a decidedly sleek look to the vulva. There is a science to this delicate process, and as one website points out, it is a marathon, not a sprint.[9] Special products are available to lubricate and shave the delicate outer skin (nowadays many men are

---

[8] https://www.nva.org/what-is-vulvodynia/vulvar-anatomy/.
[9] https://www.refinery29.com/en-us/how-to-shave-vagina.

doing the same thing [i.e., shaving body and genital hair, which can make the penis appear larger and more accessible]).

Vagina

Dr. Matthew Hoffman wrote an article on WebMD called "Picture of the Vagina" that clearly diagrams the female anatomy, including the vagina, which "is an elastic, muscular canal with a soft, flexible lining that provides lubrication and sensation. The vagina connects the uterus to the outside world. The vulva and labia form the entrance, and the cervix of the uterus protrudes into the vagina, forming the interior end."[10] "The muscular vagina receives the penis during sexual intercourse and also serves as a conduit for menstrual flow from the uterus. During childbirth, the baby passes through the vagina (birth canal)."[11]

Hymen

The hymen is a thin membrane of tissue that surrounds and narrows the vaginal opening[12] in a female who has not engaged in sexual activity or intercourse. The delicate hymen may also be missing due to some other activity or exercise.[13] The presence of the hymen is traditionally understood to be the main indicator of virginity.[14] Also called the maidenhead, the hymen is a body part that most people know little about, how it looks, or what happens to it when virginity is lost.[15]

There are actually certain cultures that are engaging in a surgical repair procedure called hymenoplasty of young women's hymens to restore their virginity in preparation for marriage.[16] Also called

[10] https://www.webmd.com/women/picture-of-the-vagina#1.
[11] Ibid.
[12] Ibid.
[13] Ibid.
[14] Oxford.
[15] https://www.ourbodiesourselves.org/book-excerpts/health-article/what-exactly-is-a-hymen/.
[16] Ibid.

hymenorrhaphy, the hymen restoration is not generally regarded as a gynecological procedure but one employing plastic surgical processes. The aim of such surgeries is to cause bleeding during post-nuptial intercourse, which is considered, in those cultures, as proof of virginity.[17]

Clitoris

Most of us know that the *clitoris* is the pleasure center of the vulva and that it doesn't have a central role in reproduction like the penis or vagina, and according to Planned Parenthood's website, it's pretty much just there to feel good. It is located under the point where the inner labia meet and form a little hood, the clitoral hood.[18] Many women who haven't located their *G-spot* that is known for "deeper" orgasms enjoy several types of stimulation of the clitoris to reach orgasm.

Medical News Today offers a detailed explanation of that most elusive part of the female anatomy in its spotlight, published in 2018, because the clitoris has long been misrepresented and misunderstood and still holds some riddles that science is yet to solve.[19]

The clitoris has three major components:

- the glans clitoris, which is the only visible part of the organ, accounting for "a fifth or less" of the entire structure
- the two crura, which extend, like brackets, down from the glans clitoris and deep into the tissue of the vulva, on either side
- the two bulbs of the vestibule, which extend on either side of the vaginal orifice

---

[17] https://www.biblegateway.com/passage/?search=Deuteronomy+22%3A 13&version=MSG.

[18] https://www.plannedparenthood.org/learn/teens/ask-experts/where-is-the-clitoris.

[19] https://www.medicalnewstoday.com/articles/322235.php#1.

(not all researchers agree that the vestibular bulbs have a relation to the clitoris, however; researchers Vincenzo and Giulia Puppo, for instance, argue that the clitoris consists of the "glans, body and crura" only.

Due to its high level of pleasurable sensitivity, the clitoris is usually the main player when it comes to the female orgasm, making it the "Grand Central Station" of erotic sensation.[20, 21]

G-Spot

Do *vaginal orgasms* exist? Can a woman achieve an earth-shattering orgasm without stimulation by any other means but a penis repeatedly penetrating her vagina? As it turns out, this is where the *G-spot* makes its somewhat tentative entrance.

Known as the Gräfenber G-Spot, after the German doctor who first wrote about it in the 1950s, the G-Spot was reintroduced in the 1980s by Dr. Beverly Whipple after she discovered that using a "come here" motion (with one's finger) along the inside of the vagina produced a physical response in women. She believed that this region could be the key to women achieving orgasm during sex.[22, 23]

[20] https://www.medicalnewstoday.com/articles/322235.php#6.
[21] Sex educator and researcher Emily Nagoski calls the female genital organ the "Grand Central Station" in her book *Come as You Are*.
[22] https://www.healthline.com/health/G-Spot-in-women#1.
[23] https://abcnews.go.com/Health/researcher-claims-spot-discovery/story?id=16204607.

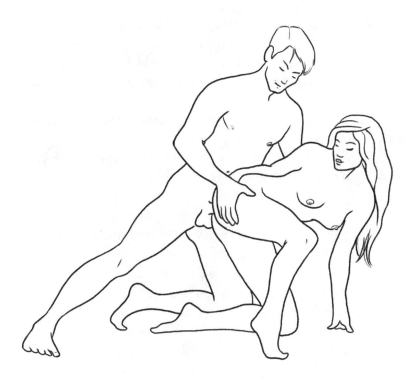

An earnest attempt to dispel the mystery about the G-spot actually points to evidence that when you're stimulating what people commonly believe is the G-spot, you're actually stimulating part of the clitoris, which is a much larger organ than so many of us, including this book's author, knew.[24]

According to WebMD, a sex quiz published online in late 2019 asserts that "whether the G-Spot exists is a matter of debate. Popularized by a 1982 book, the G-Spot is a region found behind the pubic bone that has been credited as the trigger for a vaginal (vs. clitoral) orgasm, and even a catalyst for *female ejaculation*."

However, some experts note that there's no unique anatomical structure where the G-spot is supposed to be located. If the G-spot exists, it's best described as an erogenous zone rather than a part of a woman's anatomy.[25]

But let's not end the G-spot discussion there. Other online sources elucidate further.

According to an article written by Jane Chalmers of Western Sydney University on the website Science Alert:

> The G-Spot certainly exists in some women. However, not all women will find the stimulation of the G-Spot pleasurable. Just because a woman is not aroused when the G-Spot area is stimulated, this does not mean she is in any way sexually dysfunctional. Sexuality and arousal have clear physiological and psychological links. But, as human beings, we are all made slightly anatomically and physiologically different.[26]

That same site even suggests that orgasms vary from person to person. "It is a unique experience…the complexities of human sexu-

---

[24] https://www.healthline.com/health/G-Spot-in-women#1.
[25] https://www.webmd.com/sex-relationships/rm-quiz-sex-fact-fiction.
[26] https://www.sciencealert.com/does-the-G-Spot-really-exist.

ality and the female reproductive organs mean women may achieve orgasm in multiple ways."[27]

Orgasm

While orgasm is not a part of the human anatomy, it is certainly part of the human experience, for most people (male orgasm is discussed on page 133). This is because "some women are unable to orgasm in the presence of a partner, but have no difficulty reaching orgasm with masturbation. Some women can orgasm only with clitoral stimulation, while others can orgasm through vaginal/G-Spot stimulation alone." The individual differences are extremely challenging for many people. Communication is the key here, questions and answers like, "Does this feel good? How does that feel? Do you like this?" These questions should be followed by clear responses like, "Oh my god, yes!"

> **Amusing nugget of information: In the author's experience, on the other hand, men will often blurt out the word *shit* several times when they are having an orgasm. I don't know if they're surprised or maybe disappointed that they came so soon.**

This is where I'd like to mention the website OMGyes.com, a site designed for women and their partners seeking to know all about female sexual pleasure. Available for sale in one or two sessions, OMGyes.com provides extensive, frank, and natural original video instructions for techniques to be orgasmic and multiorgasmic.

There is also an inner pleasure collection of pleasuring techniques. Ownership comes with a fairly hefty price, but women who find it difficult to orgasm will see that it is worth the investment. It even "cums" in twelve languages (sorry, I just couldn't resist).

---

[27] Ibid.

Cervix and Uterus

Most of us have seen lateral diagrams of the pear-shaped uterus with the *cervix* at its opening.[28] The cervix is also the opening during menstrual periods through which blood passes into the vagina and the outside the body. The cervix dilates during childbirth to allow the baby to pass out of the uterus and into the birth canal. During sex, the penis often bangs up against the cervix, and on occasion, this can cause discomfort in some women. But keep in mind that because the vagina is capable of expanding by 200 percent, most penis sizes can be accommodated easily.

Fallopian Tubes

The uterine tubes, also known as *oviducts* or *fallopian tubes*, are the female structures that transport the ova from the ovary to the uterus each month. In the presence of sperm and fertilization, the uterine tubes transport the fertilized egg to the uterus for implantation.[29]

Please see "Fertilization below" to learn about where the egg and the sperm actually unite.

Fertilization

Now let's address *fertilization* since it is a monumental occurrence in a woman's life that actually takes place in a section of the fallopian tube. As a sexual function, "scientists discovered the dynamics of human fertilization in the 19th century."[30] Contrary to what many people think, the egg is not sitting in the uterus waiting for those frantic little sperm to swim up the vagina and attack the egg

---

[28] https://www.webmd.com/women/picture-of-the-cervix#1.
[29] https://emedicine.medscape.com/article/1949193-overview.
[30] https://en.wikipedia.org/wiki/Human_fertilization.

there. And sometimes there are multiple eggs and, with successful fertilization, may result in multiple births resulting in twins, triplets, and even more babies. Often these babies are born prematurely, resulting in extended hospital care and the need to keep preemies in an incubator.

> Simply put, the definition of human fertilization is the union or joining of the egg and the sperm, resulting in a fertilized egg, otherwise known as a zygote. But the process of human fertilization is very complicated and comprised of many steps and components necessary to achieve the ultimate result of human life.[31]

In fact, human fertilization "is the union of the human egg and sperm that usually occurs in what is called the ampulla of the fallopian tube." The ampulla is the section of the oviduct that curves around the ovary, and it is quite a distance for the sperm to travel to reach it.

It is after this complex process occurs that "the sperm plasma then fuses with the egg's plasma membrane, the sperm disconnects from its flagellum (tail) and the egg travels down the fallopian tube to reach the uterus."[32]

It is there in the uterus, which has been prepared by the female hormone progesterone, that the egg becomes attached to the uterine wall in a state of pregnancy. "If the egg is not fertilized, progesterone is secreted by the ovaries until a few days before menstruation, at which time the level of progesterone drops sufficiently to stop the growth of the uterine wall and to cause it to break down, and menstruation ensues."[33]

---

[31] https://study.com/academy/lesson/what-is-human-fertilization-process-definition-symptoms.html.

[32] https://en.wikipedia.org/wiki/Human_fertilization.

[33] https://www.britannica.com/science/progesterone.

Menstrual Cycle

The *menstrual cycle* is the monthly series of changes a woman's body goes through in preparation for the possibility of pregnancy. Each month, one of the ovaries releases an egg—a process called *ovulation*. At the same time, hormonal changes (progesterone) prepare the uterus for pregnancy. If ovulation takes place and the egg isn't fertilized, the (bloody) lining of the uterus sheds through the vagina. This is a menstrual period.[34]

All but about 15 percent of women experience such symptoms as painful cramping, cravings, mood swings, and more for up to two weeks before menstruation that are collectively called PMS, or premenstrual syndrome.[35]

Certain religious dogma regard a woman with her period to be unclean, and even in today's world, some cultures still eject a woman during her *period* from the home to survive outdoors, even in winter weather.[36] There are varying points of view with regard to having sex during one's menstrual period. Most men, even those who are sexually enlightened, are clearly not thrilled by the prospect of giving oral sex during his partner's period but have no problem with intercourse.

The idea that menstrual blood is "dirty" because it is rejected body fluids or flushed-out toxins is a myth. In fact, it can be thought of as a vaginal secretion of some blood, uterine tissue, mucus lining, and bacteria. It doesn't affect our ability to have sex and certainly doesn't mean that conditions aren't ideal for sex.[37] However, sex

---

[34] https://www.mayoclinic.org/healthy-lifestyle/womens-health/in-depth/menstrual-cycle/art-20047186.

[35] https://www.everydayhealth.com/pms/pms-symptoms.aspx.

[36] https://www.bbc.co.uk/news/resources/idt-sh/banished_for_bleeding.

[37] https://www.healthline.com/health/womens-health/period-myths#7.

during a woman's period can be messy, indeed, requiring care not to stain bedding or clothes.

Women have to deal with a panoply of issues during their periods. About 20 percent have a condition called dysmenorrhea, which includes the debilitating cramping, anxiety, as well as diminished capacity to concentrate.[38]

I won't try to cover the entire reproductive processes such as pregnancy and childbirth for the purpose of this book, but everyone should understand how these work as part of their study of both human anatomy and the reproductive system.

---

[38] https://www.healthline.com/health/womens-health/period-myths#3.

CHAPTER 14
CHANGING SEXUAL URGES (FEMALE)

Aside from childbirth, there is nothing more challenging to a woman in her sex life than losing her sexual urges. This is usually hormonal, and depending upon the hormone levels, it can mean a range of issues between dryness and pain during *intercourse* and a complete loss of sexual desire. But wait. There is no need to despair or give up your sex life. There are solutions to these issues (see pages 141 and 270 regarding hormonal remedies [bioidentical hormones] to deal with changing sexual urges and physical challenges).

Menopause

Menopause is the time in a woman's life when her monthly period stops. It usually occurs naturally, most often after age 45. Menopause happens because the woman's ovaries stop producing the hormones estrogen and progesterone. A woman has reached menopause when she has not had a period for one year. Changes and symptoms can start several years earlier. They include:

- A change in periods—shorter or longer, lighter or heavier, with more or less time in between
- *Hot flashes* and/or night sweats
- Trouble sleeping
- Vaginal dryness
- Mood swings
- Trouble focusing
- Less hair on head, more on face[1]

Decreased Sexual Desire

According to the North American Menopause Society (NAMS), "although most women experience some changes in sexual function as they age, menopause and aging certainly do not signal the end of a woman's sex life."[2] That said, the key to whether an issue becomes a sexual problem is measured not by the problem but by how the individuals involved find it to be a problem.

If both partners in a couple are content to live without an active sex life, then a condition such as vaginal dryness or erectile difficulty does not really represent sexual dysfunction. Similarly, a woman who notices some decline in sexual desire over time may not be troubled by it if she is not in a relationship.[3]

---

[1] https://medlineplus.gov/menopause.html.
[2] http://www.menopause.org/for-women/sexual-health-menopause-online.
[3] http://www.menopause.org/for-women/sexual-health-menopause-online/sexual-problems-at-midlife.

But clearly, if a healthy sex life is desired by either or both partners, there are solutions. And these don't need to involve *sexual infidelity*, which sadly seems to be a common response to diminishment of sexual desire in both men and women (see **"There Are Solutions"** on page 115).

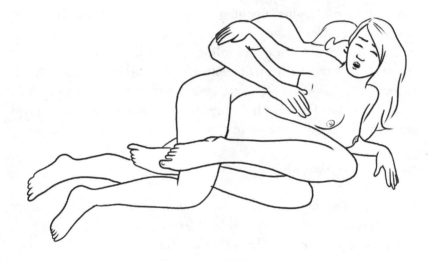

While the NAMS website provides a complete analysis of decreased sexual desire and functionality, suffice to say that the causes are complex. The upshot is that about 10 percent of US women are troubled by low sexual desire.[4] "Women's happiness with their overall relationship with their partner had an important effect on desire and any distress they feel because of low desire."[5]

Decreased Arousal

Beyond desire, "arousal involves the physical signs of sexual readiness." This involves the swelling of the labia, clitoris, and upper vagina, lubrication of the vaginal lining, lengthening of the vagina, exposure of the vaginal opening. Other changes in breathing and heart rate, muscles tensing, and nipples becoming erect; all of these indicate readiness for sex. According to NAMS, the first noticeable change associated with menopause is often reduced vaginal lubrication during arousal. Often treatment with hormone creams help with this issue. HRT or hormone replacement therapy also helps greatly with sexual desire or lubrication.

Decreased Pleasure

According to the NAMS website, a large nationwide survey about sexual behavior among older US adults, 23 percent of women, ages fifty-seven to eighty-five, said they did not find sex pleasurable. Of that group, 64 percent were troubled by this lack of pleasure. Another survey found that about 5 percent of US women have a problem achieving orgasm that causes them concern.[6] Clearly there has to be a better way.

---

[4] http://www.menopause.org/for-women/sexual-health-menopause-online/sexual-problems-at-midlife/decreased-desire.

[5] Ibid.

[6] http://www.menopause.org/for-women/sexual-health-menopause-online/sexual-problems-at-midlife/decreased-response-and-pleasure.

Pain with Penetration

As estrogen levels fall as women approach and pass menopause, the resulting dryness and thinning of vaginal tissues can cause penetration and intercourse to be uncomfortable for many women. The discomfort can range from a feeling of dryness to a feeling of vaginal "tightness" to severe pain during sex. After sex, some women feel soreness in their vagina or burning in their vulva or vagina. Over time, and without treatment, the inflammation that may result from infrequent sex without sufficient vaginal lubrication can lead to tearing and bleeding of vaginal tissues during sex.[7]

There are many factors that can affect sex drive, such as whether or not you are in a relationship, how you are getting along, body image satisfaction, dietary intake, medication use, depression or history of sexual abuse. (Lilli Link, MD, Parsley Health)

Thirteen Biggest Sex Drive Killers

Yet another list of sex drive killers.

- Stress
- Partner problems
- Alcohol
- Too little sleep
- Having kids
- Medications including antidepressants, blood pressure, birth control, chemo, anti-HIV drugs

---

[7] http://www.menopause.org/for-women/sexual-health-menopause-online/sexual-problems-at-midlife/pain-with-penetration.

- Poor body image
- Obesity
- Erectile dysfunction
- Low testosterone
- Depression
- Menopause

Lack of closeness, self-love, masturbation[8]

---

[8] https://www.onhealth.com/content/1/sex_drive_low_libido.

CHAPTER 15
THERE ARE SOLUTIONS

Take heart! Relief from all of the various forms of diminishment in sexual enjoyment that has just been discussed is available. Pharmaceutical hormonal remedies, plant-based *bioidentical hormones*, and natural herbal remedies are all readily available on the market today. We will touch on each of these here, but the emphasis will be on the bioidentical hormones because they are so highly effective and, amazingly, still comparatively unknown.

Benefits of Hormone Replacement Therapy (HRT)

A very informative slide show on the WebMD website explains that *HRT*, or *hormone replacement therapy* is designed to help with those menopausal symptoms including hot flashes, night sweats, and pain during sex because of changes in the walls of the vagina.[1] Other symptoms of menopause that have been discussed include sleep trouble, headaches, and mood changes.[2] Most of these symptoms are addressed by HRT, the various FDA-approved brands of which may be prescribed by either your primary doctor or your gynecologist.

---

[1] https://www.webmd.com/menopause/guide/menopause-hormone-therapy.
[2] https://www.webmd.com/menopause/ss/slideshow-hormone-therapy.

Hormone therapy treatment with medications that contain female hormones are meant to replace the hormones that the body no longer produces at normal levels after menopause. But it's important to know the risks involved. The Mayo Clinic website about hormone therapy indicates that large clinical trials of hormone therapy have shown health risks as well as benefits depending on the type of hormone therapy, the dose, and length of time they are taken.[3]

Risks can include heart disease, stroke, blood clots, and breast cancer. In addition to restoring sex drive, additional benefits can include treatment for hot flashes, night sweats, vaginal dryness, itching, burning and discomfort with intercourse. And even further benefits include reduced risk of colon cancer and osteoporosis.[4]

Those with a history of breast cancer, ovarian cancer, endometrial cancer, blood clots in the legs or lungs, stroke, liver disease, or unexplained vaginal bleeding should usually not take hormone therapy. It's essential to spend serious time becoming knowledgeable about the risks associated with HRT. Depending on the woman's health history, the benefits usually outweigh the risks. Talk with your bioidentical hormone doctor about your personal risks and how those risks can be minimized.[5]

Importance of Sex Hormones

An online health protocol entitled "Female Hormone Restoration," from Life Extension.com, clarifies the importance of maintaining balanced female hormones:

> Balancing hormone levels, including progesterone, estrogens (estrone, estradiol, estriol), *DHEA*, testosterone, and pregnenolone, are important for women's health. Unfortunately,

[3] https://www.mayoclinic.org/diseases-conditions/menopause/in-depth/hormone-therapy/art-20046372.
[4] Ibid.
[5] Ibid.

hormone levels in women decline as they age. Postmenopausal women are at an increased risk of several diseases, including cardiovascular disease, Alzheimer's, and osteoporosis. Menopause also often causes sleep trouble because of various disruptions of the normal menstrual cycle.

Bioidentical Hormone Therapy

The author of this book has been on bioidentical hormones since 2016 and thoroughly loves her sexuality, which has done a 180-degree turnaround from nearly 0 percent interest in sex to what feels like 1,000 percent. She feels younger, more vital, has fewer memory issues, and is as horny as a twenty-year-old. That said, looking at online research about bioidentical hormone replacement therapy (HRT) yields several outdated articles from such entities as the US government (2011), Harvard Medical School (2006), WebMD (2009), all well before this book was written (2020–2021).

> Conventional prescription hormone replacement therapy (i.e., with conjugated equine estrogens and synthetic progestin) has been shown to have serious adverse health consequences. Fortunately, bioidentical hormone replacement therapy as well as natural alternatives like phytoestrogens, may offer women safe and effective options to promote youthful hormone levels.[6]

To illustrate one of these specialized and relatively unknown products, and to harvest information about it, the hormone pellet therapy product developed by Sottopelle, the company whose bioidentical hormone product that the author uses, a brochure that is

---

6   https://www.lifeextension.com/protocols/female-reproductive/female-hormone-restoration.

packed with information developed by the Sottopelle Pellet Hormone Therapy is largely reproduced in the appendix of this book. That brochure that was given to me when I began therapy is loaded with great information about HRT, particularly bioidentical, or another term for them—bioequivalent hormones.

Sottopelle's brochure describes hormone pellet therapy as:

> A state of the art medical protocol utilizing tiny hormone pellets that provide an on-demand delivery system to replenish the missing amounts of estrogen and testosterone. They are designed to supplement or add to your own hormones—not replace them. The pellets contain low-dose, plant-based hormones derived from a naturally occurring compound found in soy and wild yam called diosgenin, which is biologically equivalent to human hormones.
>
> The pellets are slightly larger than a piece of rice and are painlessly placed beneath the skin by the doctor. This type of hormone pellet therapy allows your body to receive the balanced hormones it needs directly into the bloodstream 24 hours a day, 7 days a week.

The pellet is designed to last from four to six-month intervals. And before the pellet is replaced with a new one, hormone levels are tested at the lab.

According to that same brochure, hormone replacement therapy's benefits include:

- Increased sex drive and satisfaction
- Increased energy levels
- Increased mental sharpness, concentration, and memory
- Improves sleep
- More stable moods, less irritability and grumpiness

- Decreased body fat
- Less anxiety and depression
- Increased sense of well-being
- Increased muscle mass and strength
- Increased bone density
- Reduced night sweats
- Reduced hot flashes
- Relief of migraines

Topics such as the history of pellet use in HRT, possible side effects, delivery of treatment, and safety are all addressed in the same brochure.

A 2009 online article about Oprah Winfrey and bioidentical hormone therapy clarifies the meaning of *bioidentical* in this simple way, "Bioidentical hormone preparations are medications that contain hormones that are an exact chemical match to those made naturally by humans," said JoAnn Manson, MD, DrPH, chief of preventive medicine, Brigham and Women's Hospital, Boston, Massachusetts. Some of these hormone remedies are made by drug companies and approved by the FDA and sold in standard doses.

Others are custom-made at compounding pharmacies and are not approved by the FDA (Food and Drug Administration) specifically because they are not standardized.[7] They are custom-blended at a compounding pharmacy and shipped to the doctor to utilize with the same patient during the processes involved in this form of therapy.

That said, no warnings are provided to the patient receiving non-FDA-approved bioidentical hormone therapy because of the absence of the FDA approval process, while patients receiving FDA-approved hormone replacement therapy are provided with warnings.[8] Meanwhile, claims of increased safety of the bioidentical hormones are being argued because large-enough government studies

---

[7] https://www.webmd.com/women/news/20090115/oprah-and-bioidentical-hormones-faq#1.

[8] Ibid.

to prove the safety of FDA-approved hormones and non-FDA-approved bioidentical hormones haven't been conducted (2009).[9]

However, "Erika Schwartz, MD, a New York doctor who prescribes FDA-approved Bioidentical Hormones and compounded Bioidentical Hormones, says there have been studies that support the safety of Bioidentical Hormones, compared to other hormone therapy."[10]

As founder of the bioidentical hormone initiative, Schwartz educates physicians from around the globe on the multiple benefits and correct usage of bioidenticals despite the onslaught of money and opposition from pharmaceutical companies. According to Schwartz, hormones mixed specifically for her symptoms gave her relief when well-known FDA-approved brands of medication had not done so for fifteen years.

In an online article about bioidentical hormones published in 2011, and updated in 2018, Harvard Medical School's publishing arm concedes that:

> There actually may not be much difference between an FDA-approved bioidentical and the custom-compounded version. Both are made from the same hormones and manufactured according to the requirements of the United States Pharmacopeia (a nongovernmental authority that sets the standards for prescription and over-the-counter drugs).[11]

---

[9] Ibid.
[10] Ibid.
[11] https://www.health.harvard.edu/womens-health/bioidentical-hormones-help-or-hype.

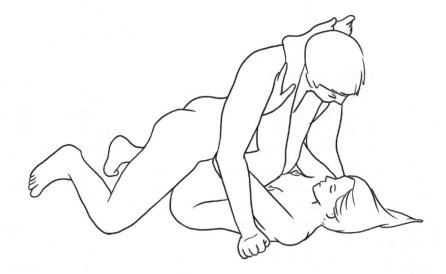

CHAPTER 16
MORE SOLUTIONS

Herbs and Supplements

Visit any large gym and check out the clientele. There are many dating-age people, dressed in cool working out clothes. Everyone's body on parade. Check into the dating sites online, you will discover that many people have largely trended not only to exercise and work out three to four times a week but also to eat more healthfully. Herbs and supplements are also usually part of their health regimen.

The following herbs and supplements are taken regularly as natural substitutes for the chemically derived medications for female sexual enjoyment, and later, you will find herbs and supplements suggested for male enhancement and erection.

Natural Female Hormone Boosters

- **Phytoestrogens**—Isoflavones (from soy) and lignans (from flaxseeds and other plants).
- **Siberian rhubarb**—Used for many years to relieve problems associated with female hormone imbalance
- **Black cohosh**—Relieves menopausal symptoms.

- **Dong quai**—Female ginseng; traditional Chinese herb used to relieve painful menstruation, menopause symptoms, fatigue, and more.
- **Cruciferous vegetables**—Like broccoli and cabbage, promote healthy estrogen metabolism because of beneficial compounds and may protect against breast cancer.
- **Licorice root**, **vitex agnus-castus**, **vitamin D**, and **fish oil** are other natural ingredients that may promote healthy female hormones.

Other Natural Solutions for Diminished Female Sexual Interest

An article[1] published in *Medical News Today* in the beginning of 2020 listed "Natural Ways to Boost Libido." Some of those include manage anxiety, improve relationship quality, and focus on foreplay because "having better sexual experiences may increase a person's desire for sex, thereby boosting their libido."

News flash: "People can enhance their sexual experiences by spending more time on touching, kissing, using sex toys and performing oral sex. Some people call these actions *outercourse*" (Zawn Villines, January 23, 2020)

Other ways to boost libido detailed in that article include exhortations to get good-quality sleep, eat a nutritious diet, get regular exercise, maintain a healthy weight, try sex therapy, and quit smoking.

Note: All of the foregoing information about boosting libido applies to men as well as women.

---

[1] https://www.healthline.com/health/boost-your-libido-10-natural-tips.

Acupuncture

According to the Acupuncture Now Foundation, acupuncture is a method of supporting the body/mind systems in their own natural healing processes. Originating in East Asia over two thousand years ago, in its modern practice, acupuncture forms a part of a rational, personalized, evidence-based system of effective healthcare. Worldwide, well over one million health-care practitioners use acupuncture to ease the suffering and restore the health and well-being of their patients. A website called Well + Good lists the benefits derived from acupuncture in boosting sex drive.

How acupuncture boosts sex drive:

- Improves circulation to help you to reach orgasm
- Helps to balance your hormones
- Relieves stress
- Reveals other issues that contribute to lowered libido

Herbs for Female Sexual Enhancement

- **Black cohosh root**—Popular treatment for women's health issues in Europe since the mid-1950s. Symptoms treated include *menopause* (particularly hot flashes), *premenstrual syndrome* (PMS), painful *menstruation*, weak and brittle bones (*osteoporosis*), and more.[2]
- **Dong quai root**—Used for menstrual cramps, premenstrual syndrome (PMS), and menopausal symptoms. Also used to manage anemia, joint pain, hypertension, infertility, ulcers, and constipation, as well as treatment of allergy.
- **Passionflower**—Used for anxiety, including before-surgery anxiety. Also used for stress, ADHD, and pain.[3]

---

[2] WebMD.
[3] WebMD.

- **Red raspberry leaf**—Used for easing labor and delivery; gastrointestinal (GI) disorders, including diarrhea; infection of the airways, including flu; and heart problems.
- **Fenugreek seed**—Used for muscle strength and weight lifting power, while possessing anticancer properties in vitro.[4]
- **Licorice root**—Used for digestive problems, menopausal symptoms, cough, and bacterial and viral infections.[5]
- **Cramp bark**—Used for cramps (menstrual discomfort, pregnancy-related cramps) and possibly lowers blood pressure and decreases heart rate.[6]
- **Chamomile flowering tops**—Used for menstrual pain, treating diabetes, and lowering blood sugar. It is also for osteoporosis, inflammation, cancer treatment and prevention, and is known especially for helping with sleep and relaxation. It also treats cold symptoms and mild skin conditions.[7]
- **Saw palmetto berry**—Commonly used in supplements to improve prostate health, balance hormone levels, and prevent hair loss in men. Other benefits include decreased inflammation and improved urinary function.[8]
- **Wild yam root**—Used as a natural alterative to estrogen therapy for symptoms of menopause, infertility, menstrual problems, and other conditions.[9]
- **Butternut bark**—Used for constipation, gallbladder disorders, hemorrhoids, and skin diseases. It is also for cancer, bacterial infections, and parasites and for use as a tonic.[10]
- **Kelp whole thallus**—Derived from fronds of underwater kelp seaweed that is prized for its iodine as well as its anti-

---

[4] Nutritionfacts.org.
[5] Nccih.nih.gov.
[6] WebMD.
[7] *Medical News Today.*
[8] Heathline.com.
[9] WebMD.
[10] Ibid.

oxidant properties. May also help slow the spread of colon and breast cancers.

- **Parsley Health**—(parsleyhealth.com) published an especially informative article entitled "Natural Herbs and Supplements to Increase Sex Drive in Women" by Lilli Link, MD, that also addresses foods to eat and avoid to enhance sexual attraction.
- **Maca**—Grown in Peru for over three thousand years; used for anemia, infertility, and sexual dysfunction.
- **Red clover**—Red clover contains isoflavones or phytoestrogens, compounds similar to the female hormone estrogen. Historically used for asthma, whooping cough, cancer, and gout. Isoflavone extracts are used as dietary supplements for menopausal symptoms, high cholesterol, and osteoporosis.[11]
- **Panax ginseng** (Korean red ginseng)—Also called Asian or Korean ginseng, Panax ginseng has anti-inflammatory, antioxidant, and anticancer effects.[12]
- **Tribulus** (*Tribulus terrestris*)—Traditionally used to enhance libido, it also is known to keep the urinary tract healthy and reduce swelling. In supplements, it is used to increase testosterone levels.[13]
- **Lady Prelox**—May improve sexual function and relieve climacteric symptoms in perimenopausal women.
- **Fenugreek**—Used for boosting testosterone and increasing milk production in breastfeeding mothers. Other applications include reducing cholesterol levels, inflammation, and appetite control.[14]

[11] Nccih.nih.gov.
[12] Online article about ginseng, David Kiefer, MD, Aafp.org.
[13] WebMD.com.
[14] Ibid.

Vitamins such as DHEA and L-arginine are recommended by a number of online sources.

There are many factors that can affect sex drive, such as whether or not you are in a relationship, how you are getting along, body image satisfaction, dietary intake, medication use, depression or history of sexual abuse. (Lilli Link, MD, Parsley Health)

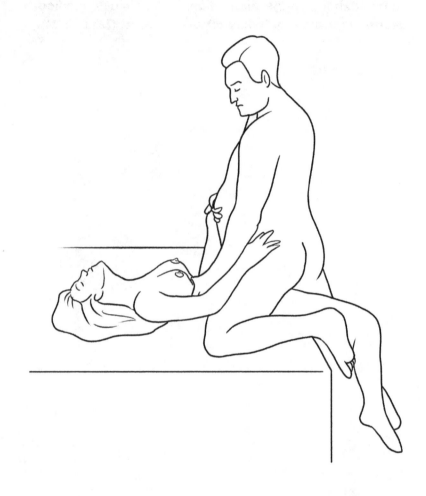

What Else Can You Do to Improve Your Bedroom Performance?

- **Give up smoking**—This is the first bad habit to go. If you fail at one method, like acupuncture, try hypnosis (or vice versa). Hypnosis worked for me.
- **Maintain healthy weight**—Eat appropriate portions of food. Don't overserve yourself. Stay away from excess fat, carbs, and sugar. Eat most things in moderation.
- **Exercise**—Walking is perfect exercise, generally speaking. If you want to accomplish other goals, such as getting in shape to have a kick-ass (weight lifter) body or to develop stamina for an active sex life, obviously specific workouts are called for as well. If you have the extra space and money to invest, you could always buy a fancy bike or treadmill. It's clearly time to become a gym rat, subject to COVID-19 safety guidelines of course.

Special Workouts for Sexual Health

Wikihow offers diagrams and step-by-step to do these special workouts for sexual health:

- Pelvic floor exercises for men—Also called the Kegel exercises for men[15]
- Kegel exercises for women—Also called the pelvic floor exercises for women.[16]

Detailed directions about Kegel Exercises may be found on the National Association for Continence website.[17]

---

[15] https://www.wikihow.fitness/Do-Kegel-Exercises-for-Men.
[16] https://www.wikihow.fitness/Do-Pelvic-Floor-Exercises.
[17] https://www.nafc.org/kegel.

CHAPTER 17
MALE ANATOMY
AND FUNCTIONS

According to Healthline male genitalia, the male genital system consists of both external and internal parts. The external male genitalia include the penis, urethra, and scrotum.

Penis

The penis is the main part of external male genitalia, which has both sexual and bodily functions. It is able to ejaculate semen (containing sperm) during sex and to relieve the body of urine. The urethra transports urine from the bladder on out of the body. Semen also travels through the urethra. In addition, precum appears at the opening of the penis, when a man is excited and ready for sexual activity.

Ode to the Penis

The uninitiated will want to learn about the immense power that the penis wields in the world. From its soft and defenseless state as a mighty organ at rest, nestled between two testes, also soft and defenseless dangling between the thighs, to as turgid as a steel rod[1] and potent in every way, to stay hard and complete sexual intercourse until release in explosive orgasmic thrusts. And if a sperm in the semen from that penis successfully travels up the fallopian tube and penetrates the egg and implants, it creates new life.

Scrotum/Testicles

Each male has two scrotal pouches, which hold parts of the internal male genitalia (epididymis, testes, and lower spermatic cords). The testes are the most important part of internal male genitalia because they make and store sperm, as well as supply the male body with hormones, which control the development of male characteristics and reproductive organs.

Nipples

Note: The author has added nipples to the list of male genitals because a man's nipples can provide tremendous stimulation. That's why it's best to ask before tweaking. Someone told me (or was it me?) about a man she knew who would ejaculate immediately if his nipples were lightly touched. A pinch would have just been too much. Who knew? This is where communication in advance comes in extra handy.

Internal Male Genitalia

The internal male genitalia include the seminal vesicle, testes, vas deferens, epididymis, prostate, bulbourethral gland, and ejaculatory duct. The testes are an important part of the male genitalia. They make and store sperm, supply the male body with hormones, and in turn, they control the development of male characteristics and reproductive organs.

---

[1] Please excuse the exaggeration.

Prostate Gland

The prostate is a walnut-sized gland located between the bladder and the penis. The prostate is just in front of the rectum. The urethra runs through the center of the prostate, from the bladder to the penis, letting urine flow out of the body. The prostate secretes fluid that nourishes and protects sperm.[2]

The prostate gland is the source of much pleasure for many men who utilize vibrators and various probe-style toys in stimulating the prostate.

This important gland can also be the source of many health issues for men to deal with in their later years. The prostate gland can become enlarged for a variety of reasons, cancer being the most serious.

Attention: The Prostate Foundation notes that there aren't early warning signs for prostate cancer (the tumor doesn't press on anything causing a sensation). That is why it is so important to get regular screenings.

Following surgery, many men experience erectile dysfunction (ED), but for most, the disruption is temporary. Nerves damaged during surgery may result in erectile dysfunction. A nerve-sparing prostatectomy may reduce the chances of nerve damage.

Symptoms of Prostate Problems

- Frequent urge to urinate
- Need to get up many times during the night to urinate
- Blood in urine or semen
- Pain or burning urination
- Painful ejaculation
- Frequent pain or stiffness in lower back, hips, pelvic or rectal area, or upper thighs
- Dribbling of urine

---

[2] Prostatecancerfree.org.

Additional Ways to Boost Libido

Other ways to boost libido include exhortations to get good-quality sleep, eat a nutritious diet, try herbal remedies, get regular exercise, maintain a healthy weight, try sex therapy, and quit smoking (these are also excellent for women).

Male Orgasm

We can't leave the topic of men's sexual features because I almost forgot the orgasm. Men's orgasms can include ejaculation or not. Ejaculation is a separate event from the orgasm. In addition, men can experience "edging" as a way to prolong a sexual experience, leaving the orgasm to the end, a culmination of physical, emotional, sexual feeling and expression. With this technique, a man is treated to a session that can last as long as an hour and involve rotating manual masturbation and oral sex.

CHAPTER 18
CHANGING SEXUAL URGES (MALE)

Dealing with Male Sexual Dysfunction

Men can have a variety of medical and some psychological issues with their genitals that are difficult to deal with, no matter when in life they experience them. These include *premature ejaculation, erectile dysfunction, low testosterone, and Peyronie's disease* (see paragraphs below for extensive definitions of each of these terms).

What Is Premature Ejaculation?

People make fun of the embarrassing phenomena technically and popularly named PE, or premature ejaculation, which is to cum sooner than planned or desired. Not only is the guy embarrassed, but his partner is usually far from satisfied.

What Is ED?

ED is the dreaded erectile dysfunction, which is a physical, and sometimes psychological inability, to achieve satisfactory and lasting erections of the penis that are so essential for successful sexual intercourse. Another term that describes it is *impotence*. The most common physical causes of erectile dysfunction are related to circulation and blood pressure. Heart disease, atherosclerosis, high cholesterol, and high blood pressure can all impact the amount of blood flowing to the penis. Diabetes contributes to ED by damaging your nerves and blood vessels.[1]

ED is often a symptom, not a condition. An erection is a result of complex multisystem processes in a man's body. Sexual arousal involves interaction between your body, nervous system, muscles, hormones, and emotions.[2]

> For many men, erectile dysfunction (ED) can be a temporary or long-term problem. In fact, approximately 52% of men between the ages of 40 and 70 years old experience ED at some point.[3]

The brain plays a key role in triggering the series of physical events that cause an erection, starting with feelings of sexual excitement. A number of things can interfere with sexual feelings and cause or worsen erectile dysfunction. These include: depression, anxiety or other mental health conditions. (The Mayo Clinic)

Popular Commercial Drugs for Male Erectile Dysfunction

- **Cialis** is called tadalafil when it's used to treat an enlarged prostate. When used as its brand name Cialis to treat erectile dysfunction, it is taken thirty minutes before sexual activity, and its effect on sexual ability may last up to thirty-six hours.[4] Cialis commonly has headache, indigestion,

---

1   Intermountainhealthcare.org.
2   https://www.healthline.com/health/erectile-dysfunction/herbs#causes.
3   "How Common Is ED," Healthline.
4   https://www.webmd.com/drugs/2/drug-77881/cialis-oral/details.

and back pain side effects. Other less common side effects include muscle ache, nasal congestion, flushing, and pain in arms and legs.[5] Cialis also has a risk of heart attack or stroke as well as other risks. It's important to become educated about all the risks involved before making the decision to use the drug.

- **Levitra (vardenafil)** and Cialis are both phosphodiesterae (PDE-5) inhibitors. That means that they work by increasing blood flow to get hard and maintain an erection. Levitra can take up to one hour to begin working, and its effects last for about four to six hours.[6] Like Viagra, Levitra also requires sexual stimulation in order to work.
- **Staxyn and Levitra** are both vardenafils, but one is not interchangeable for the other because of the strength of the dose. This medicine relaxes muscles found in the walls of the blood vessels and increases blood flow to particular areas of the body. Staxyn is used in the orally disintegrating tablet form to treat erectile dysfunction.[7]
- **Stendra** treats erectile dysfunction on an as-needed basis. Stendra also relaxes muscles found in the walls of blood vessels and increases blood flow to particular areas of the body.[8] The generic form is called avanafil. Stendra is effective after fifteen to thirty minutes, and research shows that it is effective for up to six hours.[9]
- **Viagra** normally starts working thirty to sixty minutes after you take it in oral tablet form. It may take up to two hours to work. Viagra doesn't work on its own. You'll still need to feel sexually aroused to get an erection. Used in other applications, Viagra is known as a treatment for men with ER erectile dysfunction. It is also used as a treatment for

5   https://www.goodrx.com/cialis/what-is.
6   https://www.singlecare.com/blog/levitra-vs-cialis/.
7   https://www.drugs.com/staxyn.html.
8   https://www.drugs.com/stendra.html.
9   Medicalnewstoday.com.

pulmonary arterial hypertension. Viagra is most effective when taken on an empty stomach.

Risk Factors and Side Effects

It is important to get information about risk factors and side effects, which, in each case, includes allergic reactions to the medicine. Some of these can be serious. According to GoodRX, with Cialis, there is risk of damage to the penis after maintaining an erection longer than four hours. This can cause permanent damage, including permanent impotence (the risk is rare but, nonetheless, is real).[10] It is essential to read and heed all the warnings about possible risks and side effects.

Cheaper Sources for Drugs

An article published in 2016 by CNN, "How to pay less for your prescription drugs, legally," by Susan Scutti, begins with free samples from the doctor, who gets them from pharmaceutical sales reps.

Next come generic drugs. After being on the market for a time, every brand name drug reaches a point that it is no longer protected from being copied and produced. Most drugs end up having a cheaper source and are produced with a generic name. These generics are utilized at a rate of nearly 90 percent. Despite the acceptance of generics, the prices being charged for many of them are increasing. Another issue with generics is the fact that they may vary in formulation, they may also vary in side effects. The brand name drug may or may not have more side effects than the generic.

Sometimes actually negotiating with the pharmacist for a best price may further lower the price with a larger-sized order, say ninety days, or a hardship of some sort or another, such as the poor student or the elderly person on Medicare.

---

[10] https://www.goodrx.com/cialis/what-is.

Prescription drug coupons, called eCoupons, market discounts and rebates on out-of-pocket expenses or copays directly to the consumer. Another hint to save money on expensive new pharmaceuticals is to make sure to inquire whether the generic is available. Pharmacies have to give you generic medication if you request it.

Finally there are patient assistance programs (PAPs) offered by pharmaceutical drug company programs offering free or reduced-cost medications to low-income, underinsured, or uninsured individuals. The only issue with these is the complexity of the programs' eligibility requirements, which normally includes US citizenship, some proof of income. PAP forms also require a doctor's signature.[11]

The Johns Hopkins Medicine's Patient Assistance website will find and manage your patient assistance programs. It offers access to the top fifty drug coupons.

> **You might like to take a low T-quiz online, courtesy of the Florida Men's Health Center, which offers services and information about sexual dysfunction and erectile dysfunction.**

---

[11] Ibid.

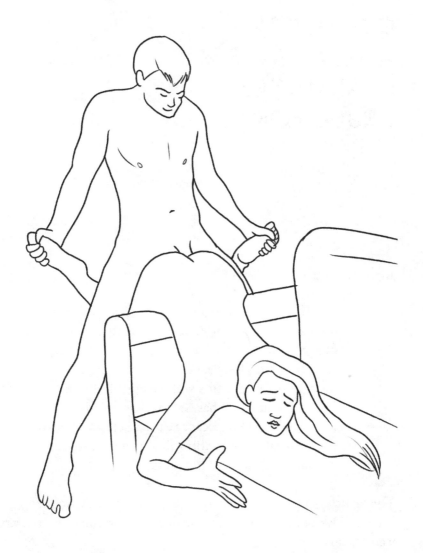

CHAPTER 19
ALTERNATIVES TO PHARMACEUTICAL DRUGS FOR ED

Acupuncture

> Erectile dysfunction is a common male disease with the constant pace of life, increasing pressure on life, and changes in diet, living environment, lifestyle, etc., lead to an increase in the number of patients with erectile dysfunction (ED). Acupuncture has been widely used in clinical trials of ED in recent years. There are many clinical trials that confirm that acupuncture can improve male erectile function.[1]

This article called "The Safety and Efficacy of Acupuncture for Erectile Dysfunction" is packed with good information you won't want to miss.

---

[1] https://www.ncbi.nlm.nih.gov/pmc/articles/PMC6336605/.

Acupressure

Acupressure is an alternative medicine technique similar in principle to acupuncture. It is based on the concept of life energy which flows through "meridians" in the body. In treatment, physical pressure is applied to acupuncture points with the aim of clearing blockages in these meridians.[2]

Healthline.com offers a clear explanation of how acupressure can work at home with self-treatment. It even offers identification and illustration of five pressure points for the treatment of ED.

Bioidentical Hormones

The Frank Institute for Health and Wellness blog published an article called "Erectile Dysfunction Treatment: How Hormone Therapy Can Help." This article asserts that "Hormone replacement therapy can actually significantly improve your erectile dysfunction symptoms." The same website offers an individualized symptom survey for men and women.

Hypnosis

Healthline has another good explanation of how hypnosis works with ED. It involves five minutes of deep relaxation, followed by "refining a focus on creating and maintaining an erection."

What Role Does the Brain Play?

In a sense, erections begin in the brain. ED can also be caused by:

- A past negative sexual experience
- Feelings of shame about sex

---

[2] "Acupressure," Wikipedia.

- The unpleasant circumstances of a past encounter
- A lack of intimacy with a partner
- Other stressors that have nothing to do with sex at all

CHAPTER 20
NATURAL HERBAL APHRODISIACS

An erection self-test is offered by Healthline to determine if the cause of erectile dysfunction is physical or psychological. This test is also known as the nocturnal penile tumescence (NPT) stamp test.

Lifestyle changes, medications, and natural or alternative treatments can all help restore normal sexual function.[1]

Five Herbs to Help Erectile Dysfunction

- **Panax ginseng**—Also called Korean red ginseng. Panax ginseng is linked to increased alertness and could potentially improve erectile dysfunction. Traditional Chinese medicine uses these supplements for a variety of reasons, including treating impotence.[2]

---

[1] https://www.healthline.com/health/erectile-dysfunction-alternative-treatments.
[2] https://www.healthline.com/health/erectile-dysfunction/korean-red-ginseng#Traditional%20Uses%20of%20Red%20Ginseng.

- **Maca**—A twelve-week study with a group of women indicated improvements in their levels of desire, with post-menopausal women reporting the most success.
- **Yohimbine**—Yohimbine is used as a dietary supplement for impotence, athletic performance, weight loss, chest pain, high blood pressure, diabetic neuropathy, and more. According to the National Institutes of Health, yohimbine hydrochloride, a standardized form of yohimbine, is available in the United States as a prescription drug for erectile dysfunction. Please note that the Mayo Clinic warns that yohimbine shouldn't be used without a doctor's supervision because of a number of side effects, including fast or irregular heartbeat, increased blood pressure, and anxiety.
- **Ginkgo**—"Best known for boosting mental power, the leaf extract of 'the oldest tree known to man' is also being used to treat impotence in men, increasing the body's ability to achieve and maintain an erection during sexual stimulation."[3] The Mayo Clinic warns that while ginkgo has the potential to increase blood flow to the penis, there's no evidence of benefit for erectile dysfunction.
- **Mondia whitei or whytei**—A medicinal plant from Africa with aphrodisiac and antidepressant properties that is used primarily for those purposes.[4]

Product Warning: Natural May Not Be Safe

The Mayo Clinic warns that

just because a product claims to be natural doesn't mean it's safe. Many herbal remedies and dietary supplements can cause side effects and dangerous interactions when taken with certain medications. Talk to your doctor before you

---

[3] https://www.webmd.com/erectile-dysfunction/news/20040505/natural-sex-boosters-gaining-ground#1.

[4] https://pubmed.ncbi.nlm.nih.gov/23039023/.

try an alternative treatment for erectile dysfunction—especially if you're taking medications or you have a chronic health problem such as heart disease or diabetes.

CHAPTER 21
ATTRACTING A PARTNER

Learn to Be Bold

This phrase is one of the top five most important messages in this entire book. And if you learn nothing else, let it be the fact that you deserve to take up space just as much as anyone else in the world. Period. Take life in bites—big ones. Devour it. If you don't take a risk and have that next experience, you may never have an opportunity again.

Banish That Shrinking Violet Part of Your Personality and Come Out into the Sunlight

When we're growing up, we are told not to expect anything specific because we may not get it, and we will only be disappointed. This made us into shrinking violets hiding somewhere in the shady parts of the garden. I say balderdash. I say, come out into the sunlight. Let it shine on you. It belongs to us all.

How and Where to Meet That Perfect Partner

When things finally get back to "normal," sometime after 2021—which we all need to acknowledge was a doozy—we can all simply go to bars, restaurants, offices and churches, mosques and synagogues and expect to meet that person of our dreams.

Me. Really? Is it that easy?

Reality. Nope, it's not.

Caveat Emptor—Three of Them

Translation from Latin: Buyer beware. Let's face it. Dating the old-fashioned way is dying out. It really is, people. If there are pretty slim pickings where you live, it may be time to go online. That said, be extremely careful about the choices you make. Meet in a safe public place for the first time. Do not send money to anyone you've met online. Always carry and use condoms. No matter what.

Flirting Online

Note: At the risk of online information becoming obsolete almost immediately, I will go into a few basic online methods and communication apps on the software market today.

- **E-mail** seems like a cumbersome way to communicate; it's been around for a long time now. Nevertheless, we continue to use it. Because it's basically safe and accepts large files. In the PC world, Outlook is at the top of the list of many e-mail application offerings.
- The **texting** app called **Messages** is a favorite communications format for mainly text messages, as opposed to graphics or pictures. It is an SMS and instant messaging application developed by Google for its Android mobile operating system. It uses phone numbers.
- **Facebook** is increasingly a site that is used to meet people. Consider these requests carefully. Do you know anything about this person? Why does this person want to connect? Do you have a friend in common? What does that friend say about this person? Otherwise it's advised to steer clear.

- **Kik** is a freeware instant messaging mobile app geared to teens and young adults who are slowly moving away from social media. It is free of charge on iOS and Android operating systems.
- **Snapchat** is a messaging app that allows users to send pictures, videos, and text messages to a selected group of recipients. What is unique about Snapchat is that the images (or Snaps) are only available for viewing for a set period of time. That uniqueness can be good and bad. There are no ways for parents to monitor behavior for possible *sexting* or to stop bullies from using it for their nefarious attacks. Snapchat can also be used to meet people by "adding" both acquaintances or strangers without their knowledge. In addition, it has a safety feature called Bark to monitor children's activity.
- **Instagram** is an American photo and video-sharing social networking service owned by Facebook and created by Kevin Systrom and Mike Krieger and originally launched on iOS in October 2010. It features Share Stories, which may be posted on one's Instagram and last only twenty-four hours. It is also a private messaging service. Browse latest trends with "Shop What You Love."
- **WhatsApp messenger**, or simply **WhatsApp**, is an American startup, freeware, cross-platform messaging and voice over IP service owned by Facebook, Inc. It allows users to send text messages and voice messages, make voice and video calls, and share images, documents, user locations, and other media (the author is a huge proponent for WhatsApp and doesn't understand why people denigrate it and treat it with suspicion. I suppose I'll learn why after this book is published). Messages on WhatsApp are end-to-end encrypted. This sounds like it might not be hackable, but I'm just not sure about that. I've been using WhatsApp for years and love it as much as you can love an app.

- **Local and long distance**—Some apps are so powerful that they can separate results by geographic location all the way down to your zip code. A friend of mine recently said, "My dream is to have my next man living in the same zip code as me." I thought that was bizarre, but when she explained that she has a powerful libido, and she would like sex more than once or twice a week, I understood why it might be expedient for the gentleman not to have to drive long distances.

  Whether to pursue someone who lives a very long drive or maybe even a long flight away is entirely up to you and depends on your current and future plans. The reason should be obvious why a distance creates a barrier that must be overcome. Why? Because you need to get together and eventually have regular sex. I mean, isn't that the object?

> **Warning: Don't think for a moment that you are in love with someone you've only met online. That is a wishful fantasy. You cannot possibly know if you are truly in love with someone until you've met them face-to-face. And even that has its limitations. And don't expect love at first sight either. Chemistry. It's a mysterious thing. It takes time to know someone. But it doesn't take much time at all to know if you are attracted.**

- **Dirty talk**—Some guys and the occasional female like to be able to verbalize during sex and convey all kinds of nasty names and commands such as "Suck it, bitch," or many others that I really don't want to promote here because I find this to be a crude and rude practice, and I don't want to encourage it by focusing on it here.

CHAPTER 22
ONLINE DATING

This is a sampling of some of the best known dating sites:

- **eharmony** is an online dating website launched in 2000. One of the original dating apps on the market, eharmony is based in Los Angeles, California, and owned by German mass media company ProSiebenSat. It was founded by Neil Clark Warren and Greg Forgatch.
- **Match**, found at Match.com, is part of **Match Group, Inc.**, an Internet company headquartered in Dallas that owns and operates several online dating sites, including Tinder, Match.com, Meetic, OkCupid, Hinge, Plenty of Fish, Ship, and OurTime.
- **Plenty of Fish** is a Canadian online dating service, popular primarily in Canada, the United Kingdom, Ireland, Australia, New Zealand, Spain, Brazil, and the United States. It is available in nine languages. The company, based in Vancouver, British Columbia, generates revenue through advertising and premium memberships.[1]
- **Tinder** is a geosocial networking and online dating application that allows users to anonymously swipe to like or

---

[1] Wikipedia.

dislike other profiles based on their photos, a small bio, and common interests. Once two users have "matched," they can exchange messages.[2]

- **Zoosk.com** features forty million singles, free to browse, and photos verified. Uses behavioral matchmaking technology to deliver better matches.

[2] Ibid.

CHAPTER 23
BEYOND VANILLA SEX

Oral sex is exotic and exciting to some people and forbidden for various reasons by others, yet it sure seems that everyone has more than just a tad of curiosity about it. The same thing goes for anal sex, which seems to be enjoying its moment in the spotlight as the most exciting sexual activity among the heterosexual demographic. Gay men are probably amused, wondering what took them so long.

Sex clubs—Having visited and participated in the sexual activity at about three or perhaps four sex clubs in New York and South Florida over the years, I can't begin to pass myself off as any kind of authority on the experience. I found being in those spaces titillating as all get out. Because? I was being watched. And? Strangers wanted sex from me. Yes? And? I guess I'm a bit of an exhibitionist. It was exciting. Those places charge single ladies very little to spend time in their club. You get a locker and a place to keep your things and, as you strut your stuff around the club, have some drinks and watch and sometimes partake in the fun activities. Jump in. It's stimulating.

Swinging—Swinging is engaging in group sex or the swapping of sexual partners within a group, especially on a habitual basis.[1] This practice often takes place in people's homes in smaller groups for more privacy. Or it also occurs in sex clubs for swingers. There

---

[1] *Oxford Languages.*

is absolutely no space for jealousy or possessiveness in the world of swinging, especially when both members of the couple play the game.

Swingers sex clubs—Usually the entrance fee charges vary depending on sex. Women usually pay a much lower entrance fee of about $20 while men pay about $100, and couples pay about the same as men. This helps to get more people in and more excitement as a result. There is no equal to the experience you have when you decide to try swinging. A swingers club called Rocalta publishes its club policies, which are a bit strict.[2]

Threesomes and more—It is not unusual for a person to enjoy engaging in sexual activity with two or more people. The more the merrier? Not sure, but to each his own once again. And of course, you must decide what sex that third member should be, a man or a woman. You may wish to try both sexes at least once. It really is a lot of fun. I can speak from experience.

Practices and Terms Used for Overweight, Heavy (Excuse Me, Fat) Women

While the fitness phenomenon is probably about equally prevalent as overweight and out of shape/heavy, in our society it follows that despite the fitness phenomenon having become much more prevalent in our society, there is a healthy percentage of younger in-shape men who actually prefer an overweight woman as a sexual partner. Nowadays there are a lot of men who are eating well, some even going so far as being vegetarian, or even vegan. But that whole lifestyle thing doesn't extend to the cougar-cub world because it just happens that many cubs prefer a more fleshy partner.

Thick is a term that's being used for the body type of an attractive (significantly older) cougar when the (much younger) cub is turned on by heavier women (don't ask for a rationale for this. I haven't heard a sufficient explanation for that behavior yet). Visit the Cougar Life site at cougarlife.com.

---

[2] https://www.rocalta.com/Club_Policies.

But like the practice of role-play, when a cub might playact that he is the young stepson, and the older sexual partner would play his stepmom, caught up in a sexual encounter together, the result can be incendiary, indeed. One of the most requested perhaps would be the master and slave.[3] The stepson/stepmother is another quintessential role-play. Visiting Wikipedia to learn about sexual role-play might open up another world of sexual games in the good sense of the word. It lists about twenty different scenarios for role-play.

> **Voluptuous, Rubenesque, curvy are elegant words for heavy and simultaneously a sexy and sensual person.**

It's a thing, people. I mean, the cougar/thick phenom. I had no idea until I entered the world of online dating myself. The acronym for women with this body type is BBW—big beautiful women. There is a growing population of guys that are as sexually attractive as any other person, yet they have this fascination for big beautiful women. You may ask, what is that like? Here's someone who can speak about BBW.

> For me, I am simply only attracted to plus size or BBW. I like women with curves, I like a woman with a big bust, bigger belly and nice hips and a large butt. It is simply what I am attracted to physically. I have always thought that a woman looks good with soft sexy curves. I like her curves accented in her clothes and protruding from her body. It is simply so sexy to me. (James L., Quora)

Proud fatty Alison Stevenson wrote an article in *Vice*, back on July 16, 2015, "How to Come to Terms with Your Attraction to 'Fat Girls.'" It is helpful in understanding the fat phenomenon. She said, "The parts of us we feel the most shameful towards just might be the

---

[3] Wikipedia.org/wiki/Sexual role-play.

very parts our partner is turned on by." She continues, "In order to end the shame that occurs on this level, women—and not just fat women—need to accept our bodies as they are."

And "Fat women are sick of being treated like freaks, and those men who are attracted to us are sick of being treated like deviants. Attractiveness exists on a spectrum, and it's time that spectrum show all of itself—rolls and all."

CHAPTER 24
THE ROLE OF PORN

Porn creates an automatic turn on for many people. It is well known that men are particularly visually oriented, which means they are more susceptible to what they see, as opposed to what they hear or feel. Of course, a soundtrack comes with a variety of moaning and sucking sounds. And nine times out of ten, a horny guy will masturbate if he is alone. So ultimately, porn does the trick, engaging three of the five senses.

Pornhub

There are many people who are into watching free online pornography, such as **Pornhub.com** You name the kind of sex you want to see, and it's on Pornhub. Some of these videos aren't as sexy as others. Some use amateurs, and others use professional porn actors. So the quality of some of it is below par. You have to pick and choose. In some googling for other porn sites, my virus-seeker blocked the entire enterprise. So be careful. Practice safe sex for your computer, tablet, or phone.

> Attention, ladies, Get your vibrator ready.
> Men, get ready to stroke. If you're together already, watch for a while, and then get busy, you two.

Personal Erotic Photography and Video

Personal erotic photography can provide endless hours of dressing up, fixing the set (maybe the bed), playing with toys, masturbating, playing with food such as bananas, grapes, strawberries, and whipped cream. This opens up a full array of topics to review.

Dressing Up

For some reason, and unless it's role-play, men aren't as likely as women to get dressed up for a sex session. For a woman, the acts of shaving her pussy (or not) using depilatory (or not), planning and getting dressed into hot sexually explicit outfits of garter belt and black stockings, thong, demibra, teddy, or see-through nightgown of lace and nylon. This speaks one language. Sex is definitely on the menu. No, sex is the menu.

That said, there's no group more into the idea of dressing up than a gay man going to a leather bar. And for a gay man, there's perhaps nothing more arousing than the sight of a well-defined masculine body dressed in leather from head to toe. There is a certain level of macho expression in these metal studded accessories and accoutrements that cannot be denied. Full leather is a turn on.

According to a review of average monthly search volumes, the results of which were followed by a survey of 1,451 participants, authoritative power roles are still all the rage. Pick up a pair of handcuffs to raise your partner's heart rate; dressing up as a police officer is the fifth most popular outfit, tied with superheroes.[1]

---

[1] https://metro.co.uk/2020/02/24/top-eight-outfits-people-want-partners-dress-sex-12291740/.

Other classics include school uniforms, firefighters, Playboy bunny, sailors, and landlords.[2]

Props and Other Things

> For quite some time, I was the mystified owner of a four or five-foot bullwhip. I'm not sure how long it was. But it was an authentic whip, for certain.

A friend who worked in the next department at a job in Manhattan unceremoniously dropped the whip in a plastic grocery bag onto my desk one morning and said, "I couldn't think of who else to give this to other than you."

I'm still not sure I know what she meant by that. After, I played with the whip a few times, mainly experimenting by gently flagellating myself and finally got bored with it and gave it away to the only person I could think of who might have a use for it. How did I know? She often wore all-black leather clothes. She and I went to the film school at NYU together for a couple of years in the early 1980s. She loved the gesture. I knew she would. I wonder if she still has it after all these years.

As far as props are concerned, I suggest adding other things to make it more exciting.

Those might range from soft rope or two to tie each other up with. Or what about a ribbon tied sexily around her neck. Both of these, especially the rope, potentially bring all sorts of spice to an otherwise plain vanilla session of sex. What about a large fur (real or faux) draped across the bed? I've already mentioned the red light bulbs.

Massage Table and Virgin Coconut Oil Lube

Get yourself a professional massage table. They fold away. Mine cost less than $150. Buy easy-care cotton flannel covers for the table

---

[2] Ibid.

and the face holder. Buy a fifty-two-ounce tub of virgin coconut oil. When you are ready, put a few large spoonfuls in a bowl and run in the microwave for a minute or so until the coconut oil is clear (warm) instead of cloudy (room temperature or cold). But be careful when applying to the skin. Test the temperature with your fingers on the inside of your wrist first. I hope that dermatologists agree that coconut oil is a great lubricant for sex, for regular massage and sexual massage. Once you try it, you may never go back to regular lube products.

> According to a 2014 study, coconut oil is also clinically proven for safe and effective use as a moisturizer. Its moisturizing properties may make the product an effective lube and allow for longer-lasting intercourse. For women going through menopause, coconut oil may be especially helpful.[3]

It's important to understand that I know of no studies have been done on coconut oil as a lubricant. And some say that it may weaken latex condoms and that lubricant should be water-based or silicone-based lubes to stay on the safe side.[4] But in my estimation, coconut oil is the perfect lube for sex.

Sexual Massage with Edging

I don't think that sexual massage is as prevalent as it could be. Often when couples engage in sexual foreplay, other things, like deep kissing and mutual masturbation, it is enough to get excited and ready for sex. But sometimes it's a great variation to start the session with a vigorous sexual massage, including quite a bit of edging, which, for a man is a mixture of masturbation, sucking, and deep-throat style of oral sex, as well as some sucking of testicles during cock-stroking.

---

[3] https://www.healthline.com/health/coconut-oil-sex.
[4] Ibid.

And of course, the requisite amount of muscle-massaging should be provided with generous amounts of warm coconut oil or some other lube to loosen up your partner. The goal of all the massaging is to ultimately massage the sexual genitalia of your partner and do it with plenty of the lube.

Dressing the Set

Maybe it is a bit tired as an idea, but still, there's nothing like rose petals scattered all over a bed to evoke the mood of romance. People are suckers for them. And of course, you have to have candlelight. Even better, buy a bunch of battery-powered imitation candles for convenience and safety. When your evening is over, you just shut them off. And if you never shut them off, no harm no foul. You can also spray the sheets with special scents like lavender or jasmine. You could set up diffusers with the same scents. If it's too much, just run them during the day before your big date. Make sure that any lights that are on are essential and very low (there's nothing like bright light to put the damper on a romantic interlude).

Playing with Toys

A bit later in this book, I will devote an entire section to toys, including vibrators, dildos, and much more. But wait, let your imagination play with your head filled with visions of dildos that come with what looks like a suction cup so you can mount it somewhere or wear it in a strap-on dildo that allows you to change the penis heads to different sizes and textures. Don't forget the lube. And don't ram your partner with a large stiff dildo or a hard penis, for that matter. That's a total violation. Lubricate it and ease it in <u>slowly and gently</u>. Slowly and gently.

Online Sex Toys

While writing this book, I stumbled over what is billed as the most complete sex online store in the universe. Adam and Eve, www.

adameve.com, also claims to be the number 1 adult toy superstore online. All you have to do is look down the list of toys that they carry, and you will be convinced that they've got all the bases covered from sex toys and dildos to lesbian bondage and masturbators. From SMBD (or *Fifty Shades of Grey* with no fewer than forty-three toys) to thirty-two different pairs of Ben Wa balls, small weighty balls that are inserted into the pussy or anus, depending upon the desired effect.

My Dildo and Vibrator Collection

I have a fairly modest collection of dildos and vibrators that I keep in the bottom drawer next to my bed. They range in size, from about three inches to nearly a foot-long electric job with heat and light. There are a lot of toys and things nowadays that don't take batteries but instead run on digital charges. Much simpler.

CHAPTER 25
MORE THINGS SEXUAL

Anal Sex

I've been learning more about anal sex lately. There are those hot men who like to have the rim of their anus licked (it's called *rimming*) and more outlandish stuff like that, all called **ass play**. Rimming, also known as anilingus, is the act of orally pleasuring the anus. This can involve licking, sucking, kissing, and any other pleasurable act that involves oral-to-anal contact. Yikes! Sorry, I just haven't evolved to that level. And I doubt I ever will.

So all of a sudden, also recently, it just so happens that I have been enjoying anal sex more frequently myself. And I found a real nugget worth digging for in an article titled "34 Anal Foreplay Tips You Probably Can't Live Without."[1] Who knew that *Cosmopolitan Magazine* had it in them? What's funny is that the article was originally called "26 Anal Foreplay Tips," and it's only recently been revised by adding eight more tips, for a total of thirty-four. The factoid below provides key information on the topic. More about this topic on pages 162 and 234.

---

[1] https://www.cosmopolitan.com/sex-love/tips/a6574/buttplay-for-the-wary/.

Factoid: The entire anal sex experience is greatly facilitated if the fuckee (the person being fucked) is 100 percent relaxed and into the whole idea. This variation isn't just for people who are straight, bisexual, and gay. It goes for everyone.

Darin Rosen at the Mega Sex Adult Emporium in Fort Lauderdale, Florida, told me that anal sex is so popular nowadays that people complain that it's hard to find a woman willing to have normal sex (i.e., vaginally).

News flash—Topic of prostate sex:

Ass play is not for everyone. Some argue that it is an acquired taste. No pun intended. However, physiologically speaking, men stand to benefit from ass play. Anal exploration can enhance both their sexual arousal and climax. The stimulation of their prostate gland makes everything more intense. A unique key to mind-blowing sex for men is the openness to explore the possibilities that comes with ass play.[2]

Of additional interest to men is the entire world of prostate stimulation. Many people are embarrassed about the idea of prostate stimulation, and this may be the first time anyone has suggested entering one's anus with any type of object whatsoever. Keep an open mind. You may just love it.

Challenge 2: Gentlemen, take yourself and your mate on a visit to an adult sex store specifically to see the array of prostate stimulation implements that are available on the market today.

Suggestion: Buy one, go home, and try it out. This kind of sex requires that you put aside all squeamish reactions to the idea of true butt pleasure. For this to work, it's critical to keep an open mind.

---

[2] Assplay.com.

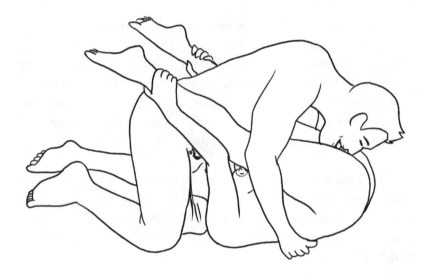

Precum and Other "New" Things

I used to masturbate with my fingers, but that is so ineffective compared to using the toys. Something else about masturbating, it should be the basis for any sexual act, meaning masturbation as foreplay is extremely effective. This is usually when a jewel of clear precum appears at the tip of the penis. Is it me or have we suddenly become inordinately fixated on precum's appearance at the penis opening? Yes, this seems to be the "new thing," like ass play is the new thing, and younger guys liking older thick women is the new thing, edging is suddenly the best selfless sex act, and so on. Yes, practices pass in and out of vogue in every major aspect of life, especially sex. We appear to be living in a very expressive time that allows us all greater latitude to express our sexuality. Anything goes!

Masturbating (Female)

One of my favorite things to do is masturbate. During the first six months of the COVID-19 pandemic, I was mostly alone and did it more than usual. I put a protective cover on my bedside chair. Next to me, I kept my choice toys and a handy small container of coconut oil. Or I'd heat a couple of tablespoons of it in the microwave for one minute to dissolve it. Usually I'd start with the glass dildo and alternate that with the nine-inch dildo and the new digital vibrator. It really helped me deal with the insanity that life had become in 2020.

Masturbating (Male)

It is well-known that men masturbate more frequently than women. It's very enjoyable to watch this or have someone else watch us while we masturbate. It greatly increases the enjoyment factor to have an orgasm while our mate watches.

Masturbating on Video (Both Sexes)

One of my online pandemic *cybersex* partners has been a guy working on an oil rig in the Gulf of Mexico. I know what you're thinking—he's a scammer. But lucky me, many contemporaneous photos and FaceTime and telephone calls have proven that to be untrue (I have rebuffed probably no fewer than twenty scammers over the three years that I have actively dated online, and I've only been burned two times for "lending" hundreds of dollars that was never returned. So I cannot and will not claim to remain unscathed by the scammers of the dating world). But I digress. Oil Rig Man made several hot naked videos and shot many cock photos—a couple of them with precome at the tip—and sent them to me. And he had so many hurricanes to deal with in the Gulf of Mexico during the pandemic that I finally realized that I will never meet him. Then the relationship died a natural death, sadly.

I meant to describe, without any visual aids, what this hot forty-something man is like. He's tall, handsome, slim, and muscular. Not like a bodybuilder; he has the solid body of someone who works very hard. He has a seven-inch-plus cock that juts out and then down when he stops playing with himself. He is fixated on the camera, as if he were making love to it. He turns around as if to display every angle of his gorgeous body. Solid. Sexy beyond belief.

> About a year ago, I shaved my pussy and took a video of a huge dildo, sliding in and out of it. Needless to say, this video has been a stellar success. (Anonymous friend on online dating sites)

Oral Sex and Gushing/Squirting

Author testimonial: This may end up on your list of TMI (too much information), but I'll go ahead anyway. Usually when a man is performing cunnilingus on me, I love for him to insert fingers inside my vagina and stroke my G-spot. That completes the feelings required for an amazing orgasm. It certainly causes me to gush liquid from my vagina during sex (that is largely due to the fact that I take bioidentical hormones). Due to the hormones, I'm able to maintain a soaking wet pussy easily for an hour or more of sex.

The Consistency of the Gush/Squirt

According to the British *Independent* newspaper, 10–40 percent of women ejaculate from their vaginas during sex (in my opinion, that is an inordinately large range. Why don't they state it this way: up to 40 percent of women?) One of the things that bioidentical hormones do for me is create the most amazing gushing liquid. I'll call it "the gush" because it doesn't squirt outward, it gushes downward. The gush yields metallic-tasting and watery in consistency, copious liquid at a warm body temperature. The wet areas on the sheets after sex are two feet across, and with a really good session, there will be two large wet areas. That's because the next layer down is a big plastic shower curtain. I'm not about to ruin a $7,000 bed.

> **Squirting and gushing—female ejaculation is not necessarily an indicator of orgasm.**

The reason I share this intimate detail with you is that I am a representative of that cohort of women who gush and squirt. In my limited experience, I can let go a stream of liquid from my pussy when I am very aroused, or when it has a mind of its own and just ejaculates. It actually ejaculates as much as a third of a pint of liquid or more in one session of sexual activity. When the woman has adequate hormone balance, moisture should be available for a hot session of sex. Men absolutely love this phenomenon. It's important to point out, though, that while ejaculating implies orgasm for a man, it is just not true under these circumstances for a woman, at least not for me. Orgasm is an entirely different outcome to sexual stimulation. For a woman, orgasm is a physical sensation and final outcome of a session of sex, masturbation, or edging. Some lucky women have multiple orgasms during a sex session. Others have only one complete one that is very satisfying.

In ancient times, Aristotle and Hippocrates pondered the origin of female sperm. It was thought that liquids excreted during orgasm were believed to have been imbued with mystical and healthful properties.[3]

If you need more natural lube in addition to a sex drive that won't quit at virtually any age, you may wish to talk with your doctor. Better yet, find a doctor whose practice is mostly *bioidentical hormones*, as I have done. That doctor is also my gynecologist.

Oral Sex Information

All kinds of handy advice about giving oral sex to men may be found, courtesy of Google, in these two articles online. The first is a recent online article from *Cosmopolitan* magazine, "45 Ways to Up Your Oral Sex Game Even More Whether You're Giving or Getting." The second, called "24 Tips for Giving Amazing Head," by Alexander Cheves, is written for gay men.

On the subject of giving a woman oral sex, "How to Give Oral Sex That Will Blow Her Mind," divulges some gems of information about the topic.

Sitting on His Face

Another oral position that is dynamite, especially if you don't have negative body issues, is sitting on his face. This just might be on every man's secret bucket list. There are those amazing men whose dedication to pleasuring his woman is when he likes her to sit on top of him with her pussy literally smack-dab on his face.[4] Frankly I don't know how those who enjoy thick women breathe while they are doing that. Perhaps they take a lot of breaks. Like cougars and cubs, it's another phenomenon that I just don't understand despite trying very hard to understand. Maybe I'll never quite get it.

---

[3] "The Science Behind Female Ejaculation," Independent.co.uk.

[4] Suzannah Weiss, "Is This the Most Empowering Way to Try Oral Sex," *Glamour Online*, June 22, 2019.

It takes a lot of confidence on the part of the woman to take the bait and agree to sit on a man's face; even better is for the two of you to decide to do it on an impulse. To me, the act of licking and kissing a wet pussy is probably measurably different from having one's face sat on. I don't know for sure. I'll have to ask some of my sexier friends. While I cannot describe it from the position of the sat-on face, I can certainly describe it from the point of view of the one doing the sitting. It's truly <u>awesome</u> (I promise to keep the *awesomes* down to a dull roar, and I think I have accomplished that goal).

CHAPTER 26
PRACTICE SAFE SEX

Rule 6: Ladies, keep different sized condoms in your purse/night table at all times. But be careful. You don't want to offer a magnum-sized condom to a guy with a small penis. And you certainly don't want to do the reverse either. If you have had even a few partners in the recent past, it's likely that you will have met at least a limited range of penis sizes.

HIV and Sexually Transmitted Diseases

Rule 7: If you are having sex regularly, especially unpro-tected sex, it is absolutely essential that you be tested for HIV and STDs. According to the clinic where I go for free testing with rapid results, the optimum testing schedule for a sexually active individual is quarterly (i.e., every three months). In my consideration, to undertest for HIV and STDs is foolhardy and to overtest is compulsive, especially if you keep coming up healthy and free of diseases. Try to keep a happy medium and practice safe sex. Use condoms. Your life depends on it.

HIV/AIDS

According to www.hiv.gov,[1] the number of people who had AIDS in 2019 was approximately thirty-eight million,[2] which is close to the population of the entire state of California. That government-generated site has an information-packed guide that takes the visitor through the process of HIV prevention, to testing, to starting HIV care, to staying in HIV care, and finally, living well with HIV. Clearly the disease is still being transmitted, which is really stupid considering that there are convenient ways to practice *safe sex*. The site is extra rich in information about HIV, including an overview of global HIV/AIDS.

> **This is a very scary fact: Approximately 1.2 million people in the US are living with HIV today. About 14 percent of them (one in seven) don't know it and need testing and treatment.**

HIV continues to have a disproportionate impact on certain populations, particularly racial and ethnic minorities and gay and bisexual men.[3]

Other Sexually Transmitted Diseases (STDs)

- **Chlamydia**—Chlamydia is one of the most common STDs. There are an estimated 1.7 million new cases a year in the US. Many people who have chlamydia do not know it. Left untreated, Chlamydia can cause infertility and pain in both women and men. Once diagnosed, it is easily cured with antibiotics. Clearly it is essential to be regu-

---

[1] https://www.hiv.gov/federal-response/pepfar-global-aids/global-hiv-aids-overview.
[2] "List of States and Territories of the US by population," Wikipedia.
[3] "Fast Facts," www.hiv.gov.

larly screened for chlamydia, especially since it often has no symptoms.[4]

- **Gonorrhea**—Gonorrhea ("the clap" or "the drip") is a serious bacterial infection of the penis, urethra, anus, throat, cervix, or vagina. Like chlamydia, gonorrhea may have no symptoms. But if there are symptoms, they can include:
  - Burning during urination or ejaculation
  - Increased greenish or yellowish discharge from the penis or vagina
  - Bleeding between periods
  - Anal discharge or bloody bowel movements
  - Itching around the anus[5]
- **Genital herpes**—According to the Center for Disease Control, the CDC, genital herpes is a common sexually transmitted disease (STD) that any sexually active person can get. Most people with the virus don't have symptoms. Even without signs of the disease, Herpes can still be spread to sex partners.[6] Most infected persons may be unaware of their infection; in the United States, an estimated 87.4 percent of fourteen to forty-nine-year-olds infected with HSV-2 have never received a clinical diagnosis.[7] There is no cure for genital herpes but medication is available to reduce the symptoms and make it less likely that you will spread herpes to a sex partner.[8] Don't hesitate to speak with your doctor about these diseases.
- **Syphilis**—One of the most serious sexually transmitted diseases is the dreaded syphilis. Easy to cure in its early stages, syphilis can have very serious complications when left untreated.[9]

---

[4] Greaterthan.org.
[5] Freestdcheck.org.
[6] https://www.cdc.gov/std/herpes/stdfact-herpes.htm.
[7] Ibid.
[8] Ibid.
[9] Ibid.

Syphilis is a bacterial infection usually spread by sexual contact. The disease starts as a painless sore—typically on your genitals, rectum or mouth. Syphilis spreads from person to person via skin or mucous membrane contact with these sores. After the initial infection, the syphilis bacteria can remain inactive (dormant) in your body for decades before becoming active again. Early syphilis can be cured, sometimes with a single shot (injection) of penicillin. Without treatment, syphilis can severely damage your heart, brain or other organs, and can be life-threatening. Syphilis can also be passed from mothers to unborn children.[10]

---

[10] MayoClinic.org.

CHAPTER 27
FLIRTING WITH PHOTOGRAPHY AND VIDEO

With the ridiculous proliferation of online dating in recent years, it's turned into an aggressive marketing job; only instead of selling something spectacular, you're basically selling yourself, and you need to be ruthless with your arsenal of weapons to use online as well as in person. Increasingly embracing X-rated photography, people are posting photos of their genitalia. This is not advisable, especially if you're using a photograph of someone else's genitalia. That would be false advertising. Don't laugh. It's true. It happens all the time.

Attention, Men of All Ages, Gather Good Photography to Help Attract a Partner

First, if you are confident, up front, and honest, you are encouraged to photograph your erect penis and save it to send it later upon request. Over my three-year online dating history, I have seen photos of probably one hundred erect penises. No exaggeration. Maybe more. I think I lost count at one hundred.

Photos for Your Profile: Dos and Don'ts

Do: Look directly at the camera lens. Smile. Show your teeth. Don't leave out the close-up/headshot. Show body in medium-length and full-length shots but not so distant that your features are indecipherable.

Don'ts: Don't wear sunglasses, especially in close-ups. Don't wear a baseball hat. Don't use group shots. And please don't stand next to or hold a dead fish (you are encouraged, however, to stand next to a sloth, which I saw on an online dating site). Don't stand with your hot rod car or motorcycle. Don't take numerous shots of the exact same angle of your face with different clothes. Don't use shots of you that are so distant that your face isn't visible. Avoid the use of the words *easygoing* or *down to earth* or *laid back* in your profile. I did a casual survey on a couple of dating sites and found that approximately nine out of ten men use at least one of those words to describe themselves to potential partners. Time for a little originality, guys. Clearly the entire country is virtually so laid back or down to earth that he'll miss the relationship boat. Men! It's time to man up and be aggressive about what you want. Make her feel really special because you took the time to get to know her. Treat her like the fascinating individual that she is.

Ideas of photos for women to take—Sexy shots: (1) Headshot with seductive makeup with red lipstick and dark eyes and hair tied up high on head; (2) Shot of entire body including high heels and complete seductive makeup and sexy black seductive outfit. Suggestions: Low-cut black teddy. Black lace garter belt with attached black stockings with lace tops, lace black thong underpants, demibra (with partial cups that don't quite cover the nipples and act as a shelf for her breasts), a sexy thin black ribbon wrapped around the throat and tied in a bow. Make sure you put on the stockings and garter belt first. Then your panties, for obvious reasons if you think about it. That way, you can leave the garter on after removing your panties.

News flash: Some women prefer a smaller or average-sized penis because their own bodies are on the petite side. Or they may prefer a smaller penis for oral sex because there is less chance to choke from lack of air (Joke? Nope).

Ladies, this is a good thing.

Gentlemen, this is a good thing. But if a woman can't take any cock in her mouth, that's not a good thing. Patience is a virtue.

Challenge 3: Ladies, practice your oral skills on a small-sized pliable dildo first. Start small and move up as you acclimate yourself to it. Learn to breathe rhythmically between strokes. All you need to do is suspend breathing for a split second. Relax. Eventually you will be so comfortable that you will want to do it every time.

Gentlemen, I suggest that you just relax and let it happen. Tell her when it feels great. She'll keep doing those things for you.

Erotic Photography and Video

The world has indulged in erotic images since man first chiseled nude statues in Greece and Italy. The massive nude statue called *David* was finished in 1504 by Michelangelo (I seem to recall that David had a very average-sized penis). Then in the late 1500s, early 1600s, there was Flemish artist Peter Paul Rubens, who loved his women on the, shall we call it the *Rubenesque* side. Considered one of the most influential artists of the Flemish Baroque tradition, Rubens was commissioned by King Philip IV of Spain to paint over eighty works. These and many other artworks executed during the Renaissance and Early Modern periods of art are still influential in our lives today. I am mentioning this because the sheer volume of erotic photographs and video that exist in this world today boggles the mind. And so much of it is online.

Every shot, each video has the potential to be art when you are memorializing the human body. That said, you and your subject(s) might want to keep an open mind to the idea of selling excellent artistic images. Or you could collect images made from live experiences. Or you could make sets of your own albums, especially for any *swinger* friends that you might encounter.

What photographs should you take? Any of the naked body that float your boat. Use props like toys and lube. Use a bubble bath or a whirlpool bath. Use special lighting. Ladies, wear hot seductive makeup. Red lips and dark eyes. What about fur throws, piles of pillows, and what else?

A friend of mind made a video of her increasingly wet pussy as she was thrusting a large dildo in and out of it until she had an orgasm. It's a short video, but that thing was so hot. Yes, I have to say it again, it was awesome.

Other hot videos may be made when sexy clothes are part of the scenario. It doesn't have to be stockings with garter belt, thong panties, demibra, and hot teddy, but it certainly could be. Variations might include strategically draping fabric on the nude body. A hot gay shot might include a nude man with his genitals all hidden tightly in a pouch G-string. Or an erect cock in a hefty *cock ring* or penis ring. That will get attention. Many hot ladies like to wear sexy shoes. We used to call them our Joan-Crawford-fuck-me shoes. Crawford wore amazing platform pumps in her 1940s movies.

Now you more than understand how endless the possibilities truly are. Having your partner take the shots or the video makes it that much hotter. Just let loose and express yourself. You don't need expensive equipment. A smartphone is really all you need. Let your imagination rule the night. Have fun.

The Pill-Swallowing Test

This is a reliable way to find out if she can give a good blow job. Give her a glass of water and a large pill or capsule of whatever she takes normally, such as a nutritional supplement or a painkiller for a headache. Watch closely how she takes that single capsule. If it's a big job for her with much gesticulation and squeamishness, stop the bus. She will probably give horrible blow jobs. She's doubtless phobic about choking.

There's nothing more desirable than a person who truly adores sucking cock, loves to deep-throat an erect cock, loves to stroke cock while sucking on testicles. And so much more. A woman who just can't bring herself to do any of these things is clearly missing the sexual boat. Use your imagination. Let it run free. Oral pleasure is the best most intimate sexual activity. To deny a sexual partner's desire for oral expression is a shame, indeed.

A woman I met at an HIV and STDs clinic inside a thrift shop benefitting HIV and AIDS in Wilton Manors, Florida, admitted that she couldn't give her husband a blow job because her extreme gag reflex prevented it. The couple had been married for eighteen years. She told me she couldn't possibly swallow even a pill without all kinds of machinations.

Ass Play

On *Urban Dictionary, ass play* is defined as "stimulating some-one's anus with any of the following: finger, mouth, toe, fist, hamster, cell phone (set to vibrate)." I'm sure it's meant as a joke, but some things in life shouldn't be jokes. I must go on the record and disagree with at least a couple of those items at the end of the list, even if they are only meant to be amusing, because they are downright dangerous.

A gay friend of mine called me from the ER recently. He said he was there for something really embarrassing. He'd been trying to stimulate his prostate by entering his anus with a small toy, which was out of reach and lost in his rectum. When he arrived at the ER, he was reassured not to be embarrassed because it's something that happens to a lot of men. That's because the prostate gland is a man's best friend. I guess you could call it man's version of a clitoris.

There are also *butt plugs*, made in graduating sizes to (learn to) enjoy something smooth slipped into the rectum and to increase the capacity of the rectum. When you get into rectum play, you'll realize what you've been missing. For some people, butt plugs are just a regular sex toy.

Ass play seems to be gaining in popularity since it is increasingly requested by men my friends and I date, even though—I am sorry to admit—I have shied away from it in the past for the most part. But after making it a point to try certain things out, I am finally ready to announce that I've joined the ranks of the ass play generation. Now I even get a hankering for anal penetration during hot sexual activity. I've been talking about it with several people lately, and they all notice the same increase in ass play. I find it amusing that people would choose this to be a new and focused pursuit over any others. Go figure.

Prostate Orgasm

In keeping with the ass end of things for a while longer (pun intended), Healthline.com offers a great guide in an extensive article called "How to Have a Prostate Orgasm: 35 Tips for You and Your Partner."[1]

Highlights: The prostate or P-spot is a small muscular gland that produces the seminal fluid found in ejaculate and helps propel semen from the penis. It is also surrounded by nerve endings that can feel oh-so-good when touched just right. But only *cisgender* men and people assigned male at birth have them.

The prostate is located about two inches inside the rectum, between the rectum and the penis. Being aroused causes the prostate to swell, which makes it easier to feel. Prostate orgasms are more intense (than penile orgasms) and felt throughout the entire body. "There are reports of people having super (prostate) orgasms, which are a stream of fast, continuous orgasms that cause the body to shudder." Sounds pretty awesome to me.

> **You can reduce the risk of infection by changing condoms and washing well. You should never go from anus to vagina or mouth without washing with soap and warm water completely first.[2]**

---

[1] https://www.healthline.com/health/healthy-sex/prostate-orgasm.
[2] https://www.healthline.com/health/healthy-sex/anal-sex-safety#how-to-practice-safe-sex.

Healthline also features an article online called "Anal Sex Safety: Everything You Need to Know." It acknowledges that despite the fact that (anal sex) is a bit of a taboo subject, it is also an increasingly popular sexual activity, especially when it comes to couples under forty-five. A national survey revealed that 36 percent of women and 44 percent of men have had anal sex with an opposite-sex partner.

Breasts/Breast Man

Men and women alike obsess about big breasts. Men want to suckle at them. Women want to flaunt them. Mammary glands meant for a baby turn men into big soft babies. It's a good thing, guys. Ladies, you know you love it. Men who are totally obsessed with breasts are called breast men. What else can we say about breasts? There are certainly a lot of slang names for them. Something like forty-five. Here are just a few:

- Tits
- Boobs
- Titties
- Jugs
- Chi-chis
- Mammas
- Knockers

There's no doubt that breasts have tons of sex appeal. Straining under tight fabric, round, bouncing, pendulous, busting to get out. Innately satisfying handful of flesh. Much less the nipple sucking fascination so many people have.

Sexy Lingerie and Clothes

Sex is largely a visual urge, especially for men. A hard-on is quickly achieved at the sight of his partner dressed in revealing black teddy with thong panties and garter and stockings. And if you let your imagination out to play, there's no limit. Naturally the sexual imagination is nearly limitless in the store in Fort Lauderdale, Florida, called Hustler Hollywood. Does the name Larry Flynt sound familiar? If it does, you're probably old enough to recall what happened to this controversial figure in the X-rated world who published the *Hustler* newspaper. Okay, back to sexy lingerie and clothes.

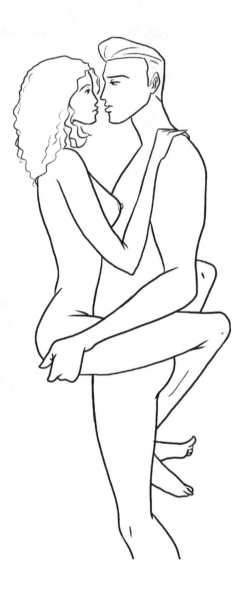

There are so many different sexy outfits that people can wear for their sex play sessions. There are clothes for a broad range of role-playing combinations, including switching your normal roles (i.e., dominant and submissive). If you like to assume different roles and wish to try more, visit your local sex toy and fashion store for ideas aplenty.

Check out the bestlifeonline.com site for basic information about anal sex, including toys, tricks, and tips to making it as pleasurable as possible. Another great information site is Volonté by LELO.[3]

Muted Lighting

The role of muted lighting cannot be emphasized enough. It automatically creates just the right atmosphere. It doesn't have to be limited to the low setting of three-way bulbs (although that is a good solution). You could also use faux candles with battery power. Probably the least desirable way to create atmosphere is with wax candles because of the obvious danger entailed in fire with unpredictable sexual activity.

Music

I'm a fan of R & B (rhythm and blues) and soul. It was ingrained in me during my freshman year in college. What heady times those were. In my opinion, music like this is very conducive to sexual activity. Soft jazz and classical music choices might include Ravel's "Bolero" or Tchaikovsky's "1812 Overture" or Beethoven's "Moonlight Sonata," or my favorite, George Gershwin's "Rhapsody in Blue." Obviously music is such a personal choice that it's absurd to even try to address it in detail here. All I can say is, let it be one of the questions you ask of each other when first meeting. If she hates country music, and he plays it all the time in his car, Houston, we've got a problem.

---

[3]   www.lelo.com

CHAPTER 28
COMMUNICATION IS THE KEY TO SUCCESSFUL SEX

The Crucial Conversation about Sexual Preferences

It's always a good idea to establish certain things before you have sex with your partner for the first time. These are not sexy seductive questions. They are:

1. Have you been tested for HIV and STDs within the last three months?
2. What types of sex are planned? (A) Oral, (B) rectal, (C) vaginal, (D) combination
3. Do you have the proper types of condoms, *dental dams*, etc. to practice safe sex?

The First Sex Questions That Many Men Ask

- **Where can I come? Or where should I shoot my load?**
  I feel certain that those two represent the most-asked question in the online dating world. Men seem obsessed with it. Is it about being polite with some advance notice?

I like to say, "All over my face and in my hair," or "Let me smear it all over my breasts. I love it. I'm not squeamish."

- **Do you swallow?**

     Swallowing fast in order to say, "Absolutely." According to Healthline, "Studies show evidence for the natural antidepressant properties of semen; some believe it could also have stress-relieving properties." This claim is due to the mood-boosting properties of oxytocin and progesterone hormones, the both of which are found in semen. Please note that practicing safe sex does not include unprotected oral sex.

- **Do you have a tight pussy?**

     He might be asking this because he's not so well endowed. So if a woman has a tighter vagina, perhaps from never giving birth vaginally, it might be a more pleasing sensation. For those who need Kegel exercises (for men and women), visit the National Association for Continence. These exercises are used to strengthen the pelvic floor, which aids in everything, from better bladder control and reducing overactive bladder symptoms, and better sex.[1]

- **How big are your boobs?**

     There are very few straight men who are not obsessed with breasts. Many of them suck on them to stimulate their partner. Enough said. It's important to point out that breasts are well loved by other sexual persuasions. Some people are into suckling like a baby, especially when engaged in role-playing. Others tweak nipples for stimulation. Still others like the sensation of having the nipples squeezed with clamps. And much more.

---

[1] https://www.nafc.org/kegel.

Questions for Ladies to Ask

Ladies! It's your turn to ask him the probing and inappropriate questions.

- **How large is your cock?**
  Choose one: Average isn't bad at all.
  While "average" for a penis length sounds like nothing much, most guys around six inches call themselves average in the US. According to Boston Medical Group, a "worldwide review of studies found that, on average, a normal penis is 3.61 inches in length when flaccid and 5.16 inches in length when erect. Average girth is 3.66 inches when flaccid and 4.59 inches when erect."[2]
- **Haven't measured it**
  Bull Pucky. He's just trying to minimize the importance of his length and doesn't want to let on that it really matters greatly. He knows exactly how long it is. Every inch. Every half-inch. Every single—oh, forget it already, won't you? I don't have proof of this; I just think that I'm right. I guess I should expect protest letters. I'm not sure.

- **What school did you go to?**
- **What do you do for a living?**
- **How educated are you?**

These are the money questions. He or she is probably looking for a spouse and knows that education and occupation speak volumes about that person's future. Even down to the school that a person attended (i.e., was the school an elevated Ivy League institution like Harvard or Yale, or some online course he/she took online at the other extreme). It's a good idea to find out if you're attracted to

---

[2] https://www.bostonmedicalgroup.com/whats-the-average-penis-size/.

someone who only has a high school education, and you have degrees. That may make communication difficult.

- **How tall are you?**

   Body statistics speak volumes about a person. For me, at 5'5", the optimum minimum height of 5'10" (for men of course) and proper weight control both usually spell success in life.

   A research paper published in the Journal of Applied Psychology showed that height is strongly related to success for men... The researchers found that on an average an increase in height by one inch at age 16 increased male adult wages by 2.6 percent.

Wikipedia does a good job in explaining how both men and women care about height.

CHAPTER 29
WHAT TO DISCUSS: IMPORTANT TOPICS

Types of Sex Preferred

HE. (A) Definitely a full blow job and first hard-on, and when I recover and can get hard again, a great fuck from behind.
SHE. (B) I'd love oral sex and intercourse in the missionary position.
Translates to:
HE. (A) Not looking for intimacy. Instead, want hot impersonal sex. May wish to "go down."
SHE. (B) A man who gives good oral sex is worth his weight in gold. Takes sex way up the intimacy scale.

In order to avoid the kind of thinking that was just described, when people are still in the early stages of a relationship, they need to establish **the style of intimacy**, the whole shooting match for how the relationship will proceed. Share decisions between you. And it's a good idea to keep track of the outcums. Of course I mean *outcomes*, but I couldn't resist.

Kissing has a huge part to play in the kind of intimacy we seek when we're developing a deeply satisfying relationship. There are a number of forms of kissing that are only incidental, such as a peck on the cheek or the lips or an air kiss. But the kind of kissing that we are talking about here is deep tongue kissing, also called *French kissing.* Okay, everyone, this is a huge germ exchange. You just can't escape that fact. That certainly makes it extremely intimate. And let's face it, sex is a messy enterprise.

Nipple stimulation is very important for most women, but less so for men. According to Healthline, men's nipples are sensitive to the touch and come in handy for erotic stimulation.[1] Nipples are a huge erotic business with clamps, clips, nooses, piercings, and more being employed for sexual nipple stimulation supreme by both men and women. What man can resist the impulse to be cradled in a woman's arms and suckling her nipples while gently squeezing and massaging her breasts. This is a key turn on for men during role-play sessions. This one is the most popular among the hot stepmother-son couplings.

Oral sex, blow job or fellatio—*Oxford Dictionary* defines *fellatio* as oral stimulation of a man's penis. It is also commonly known as a **blow job, cock sucking, giving head, sucking dick,** and many more.[2] Fellatio is sexually arousing for both participants and is highly effective foreplay for other sexual activities, such as vaginal or anal intercourse. The sex partner may be of either sex.

When people have trouble performing fellatio, they usually have sensitivities to the natural gag reflex. Fortunately it is possible for people to learn to suppress that reflex. And for the person performing fellatio, the act of giving oral sex to a man is an enormous turn on. This provides the makings of a blow job or edging enthusiast, where the idea of giving becomes even more appealing, at certain times, than any other kinds of sex.

Give Nothing but Pure Pleasure

This is the moment you enter the zone that is the purpose of this book. The rewards are plentiful when you realize

---

[1] https://www.healthline.com/health/mens-health/why-do-men-have-nipples.
[2] https://www.powerthesaurus.org/fellatio/synonyms.

your power to give nothing but pure pleasure. Pardon the tendency to hyperbolize here, but seriously, this is the mantra for my book, "Give nothing but pure pleasure." I'd love to see that on needlepoint pillows all over the United States a year after this book is published. But don't make embroidery your main activity, if you catch my gist.

Obviously the same thing goes for the woman receiving that kind of pleasure orally in direct contact with the vulva. There is nothing to compare with great oral sex. *Oxford Dictionary* defines cunnilingus (oral sex) as stimulation of the female genitals using the tongue or lips (I'd suggest to the *Oxford* people that they might want to change that to read tongue *and* lips. I don't know about you, but I'm a member of the all-or-nothing school of thought.

Another definition comes from Wikipedia about cunnilingus suggesting that tongue and lips are just the beginning and that the giving partner should also employ his/her nose, chin, and teeth. "Movements can be slow or fast, regular or erratic, firm or soft, according to the participants' preferences."[3] And obviously, or perhaps not so much, the arousal level of the pussy being eaten will decide the level of pressure being applied. Let's face it. If she's moaning for pleasure, you're doing something right.

The unfortunate truth is "people may also have negative feelings or sexual inhibitions about giving or receiving cunnilingus or may refuse to engage in it."[4] And as far as I'm concerned, this isn't just unfortunate. It's a downright crying shame, that's what it is (I am convinced that with the proper washing of the genitalia, there should be nothing objectionable about oral sex and human sexuality. Of course, all of this presupposes the total absence of sexually transmitted diseases, such as HIV and STDs.)

---

[3] https://en.wikipedia.org/wiki/Cunnilingus.
[4] Ibid.

Intercourse (the Polite Formal Way to Say Fucking)

This is generally referring to the penis-into-vagina type, for the purposes of this book, but also can include oral and anal.

> Double standard? Some men think that they can venture away from his marriage enough to have a woman perform a blow job without consequences, as long as he stops short of actual intercourse (lovemaking) which, in the author's opinion, is full-on cheating. Is this true for you and your partner?

CHAPTER 30
PREFERRED HETERO
SEX POSITIONS

Doggy style is the most popular sexual position for intercourse. After that cum (sorry, I just couldn't resist) missionary and cowgirl.[1] The position for the female is to lean on her hands or elbows or all the way down, with head and shoulders pressed down on the bed, and her knees, thus presenting her ass to the male for tipping up for regular pussy-fucking or, more directly, for ass play or anal intercourse.

Missionary position seems like a misnomer for a position that gives so much pleasure with face-to-face full-frontal exposure and ample opportunity for other kinds of intimacy, including deep kissing and caressing.

"Missionary sex simply means that the person doing the penetrating (whether it's with a penis or a strap-on) is on top and the person receiving is lying underneath them."[2] The reason it's called missionary sex is that it is the simplest position for pregnancy and accepted by observant religious people who eschew other types of

---

[1] https://www.womenshealthmag.com/sex-and-love/a19970904/most-popular-sex-position/.

[2] https://www.womenshealthmag.com/sex-and-love/a19917201/missionary-sex/.

sex. Wikipedia has some interesting material on missionary sex. Just google it.

"Missionary sex can be hot because of the intensity it can bring on—the skin-to-skin contact, eye contact, the close-up smells of each other's bodies, and just the mere closeness of two bodies," explains Debra Laino, DHS, a sex therapist and professor at Jefferson University and Wilmington University.[3]

Cowgirl position is an easy-to-perform woman-on-top position that isn't gender exclusive (that said, we will demonstrate with a man and a woman and explain from the POV of the female on top).

With the man lying on his back, straddle his hips and position yourself over his penis. Hold his erect penis in one hand and slide down onto it. Smearing it with some lube beforehand will add to your pleasure. The key element of this position is not to sit upright on top of him, but to lean forward over him, which means you can use your hands to support yourself, either placing them on his hips, or either side of him. When you're in the position, you can swivel your hips like a dancer, bounce or grind on him and control the depth and rhythm of your thrusts.[4]

In the cowgirl position, the female has complete control and can dictate the rhythm, pace, and depth of penetration. It is one of the few sex positions that allow the female to look down at the male; it's a position that strengthens a sense of intimacy, as well as being very erotic. Women are more likely to achieve orgasm in this position.[5]

---

[3] Ibid.
[4] https://www.netdoctor.co.uk/healthy-living/sex-life/a33010894/cowgirl-sex-position/.
[5] Ibid.

According to *Cosmopolitan Magazine*, angle is everything. Mayla Green, sex expert and cofounder of TheAdultToyShop.com, suggests that instead of creating a ninety-degree angle for the cowgirl position, you lean forward slightly (up to a forty-five-degree angle) for the easiest and most comfortable penetration.

Another sex expert says to vary the speed and depth of penetration so there's no discernible pattern. "Start with shallow, fast thrusts, and let yourself slowly fully sink onto your partner every fifth thrust," said Alicia Sinclair, certified sex educator and founder/CEO of the Cowgirl, a vibrating machine for women providing stimulation of the vulva, the vagina, and G-spot.

> **Wistful note from author:** I wish that I were still this pliable.

Variations

While I do love sex positions galore, I have a feeling that we could get a bit bogged down with all of them here. I will discuss a couple more in this book but suggest that if you're interested, you should do further research into all the sexual literature that you can find, from the Kama Sutra on up. I even suggest the brilliantly written and very evocative erotic classics of the Marquis de Sade. *Justine*, *The 120 Days of Sodom, Florville and Courval* are all amazing stuff. Very sophisticated.

Standing—While it certainly doesn't float my boat, standing upright offers another group of (precarious perhaps) positions that, despite not being physically easy, offer some serious variation to your sex life. *Health Magazine* offers a perfect article called "The 5 Best Standing Sex Positions."[6] Well, yeah. I guess.

Prone bone—This recumbent (flat on a surface) position is like doggy style, and with the prone bone, it "hits the G-spot with ease. It also makes the penis go much deeper so she feels all your fullness."[7]

---

[6] https://www.health.com/sex/standing-sex-positions.
[7] https://allstarpositions.com/prone-bone-position/.

Safe word—Agreeing on a safe word is an important aspect of communication before sexual contact. Definitions.net defines *safe-word* (noun) as a word used in *sadomasochistic* sexual practices to indicate that a participant wants to stop. This may be due to anything, from discomfort to out-and-out pain. That said, people seem to have very divergent reactions to pain inflicted during sex. And occasionally, a person can be less sensitive to such discomfort because they are particularly aroused during sexual activity (but please note that this does <u>not</u> give you license to compromise a person's safety in any way during any kind of sexual activity). I firmly suggest that any activity that leaves welts on your partner's body is an inappropriate activity. That goes for welts and imprints from ass-slapping or spanking and more, like hickeys on the neck, which some people wear as a badge of honor after a hot night of sex.

CHAPTER 31
NOW WE'RE
GETTING JUICY

Spanking—Often people seem to gravitate toward spankings, either given or received, with a higher degree of sexual excitement. But degrees of pain must be low and care be given to make sure this is the case because if it is too painful, that too, might cause the sex act to come to a screeching halt. And we certainly don't want that to happen. As one who likes spankings myself, I would like to offer here to the effect that I don't want your hand imprinted in red on my poor ass for days later. It's best to start soft and work up more slowly to the harder spankings. Besides it's very exciting during vigorous sex, just as exciting as hair pulling.

Hair-pulling—Really a subset of BDSM activity, hair-pulling is a big turn on for women while they are being fucked. Warning: This activity is best performed with a woman who has long thick hair. If her hair is thinner, she probably won't go for it. It's best to pull hair collected in a ponytail because it's the entire head of hair. The best image of hair pulling I can suggest is from behind during doggy style sex, or anal. How's that for playing subjugation? Anal sex and hair-pulling. Wow. More information about anal sex may be found at www.bestlifeonline.com/anal-sex-guide/.

Dominant—According to yourdictionary.com, exploring the word *dominant*, there are numerous definitions and ways in which the word is used that it will make your head spin. For our purposes, it technically means the dominating partner in a sadomasochistic sexual activity. I also found a declaration on the Insider.com website about domination, "We must be fair, things must be equal, we must take care of the other person, we must make sure everyone else's needs are met before ours." I have to say, that statement seemed a bit foreign to me at first. But the irony is not lost. I say that everyone must agree to abide by those precepts, even while using sadistic and masochistic sexual methods with their partner. If that is even humanly possible in the first place. I certainly hope that it is.

Submissive—The opposite of dominant, the term *submissive* does not necessarily mean that you are a bottom, which is the one on the bottom receiving during sexual intercourse. People who engage in submissive sexuality often fantasize about it for a long time before trying it. In real life, sexual *submission* is about control. Before you start, decide together what sexual roles you want to assume during the *role-playing* part of the fun.

Role-playing—Men are often very imaginative with their role-playing/sexual acting out activities. This is because they have the experience to know what turns them on. Whether it's the stepmother-stepson combo (a classic), the teacher-student combo, the French maid, the combinations go on and on. You can purchase many imaginative costumes from your friendly sex clothes and toy store.

Fetish—I was approached on a cougar-cub site recently by a guy who explained that he had a fetish about role-playing with partners who would agree to be his mother in an elaborate scenario, which he had to act out completely to have his best orgasm. *Oxford Dictionary* explains that a fetish is a form of sexual desire in which gratification is linked to an abnormal degree to a particular object, item of clothing, part of the body, etc. Other words that are similar in meaning to fetish: *fixation, obsession, compulsion, mania.*

Rope—Another *bondage and discipline* tool. It's best to buy soft rope because it doesn't burn the skin when it's tied fairly tightly.

Experiment. Spread-eagle is good. But some prefer to bind ankles together. Just be careful please.

What Have I Left Out? Foreplay

How could I? It's such an important tool in your sex toolbox. It's the one that women always seem to need so much, but they must rely on their man to perform it. They often complain that they don't get enough of it. Starting with deep kissing and caressing, foreplay is best when it starts slowly and becomes more deliberate as the excitement builds. Kissing the neck and breasts, concentrating on the nipples comes next. As she is more aroused, it's finally time to move on down to perform some oral sex. Then, and only then, if she has any say in the matter, it is time to move in for actual intercourse.

Ladies, it's your turn to show what you can do. Some nice cock-sucking or position 69 for mutual gratification are popular suggestions.

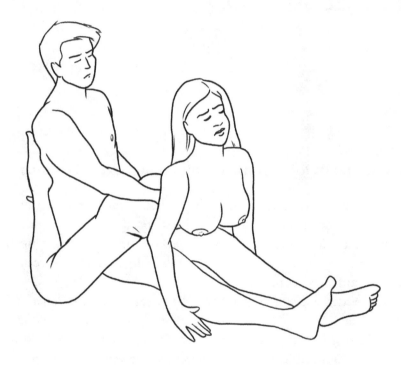

CHAPTER 32
SETTING THE SCENE FOR SEDUCTION

Preparations for Maximally Enjoyable Sexual Sessions

There is nothing more inviting than a bed set up for seduction on a romantic occasion. Of course, red rose petals come to mind. But that's so obvious and unoriginal. Why not at least change up the color of the rose petals and include petals from other soft flowers, like white gardenias, complete with their characteristic fragrance. The heady gardenia is so pungent with soft sweetness that it demands to be noticed.

I do something practical before anything else with the bed. I cover a king-sized bed with a large plastic shower curtain to prevent damage to the bed from body fluids resulting from sex. Then I cover that with a fitted sheet and place pillows at the headboard and a fluffy white fur thrown over the bottom of the bed. Voilà. Now you have a perfect playground for a hot session of every kind of sex. I guess my Girl Scout preparedness training is finally paying off.

Of course you should get out the various sex toys you anticipate using, and plenty of lube. Those can be laid out near the bed, all ready to use. If you're using extra virgin coconut oil, it makes sense to heat it up for about a minute in the microwave and place it on a towel to catch the inevitable drips. The melted version is far better because it is smooth and sleek and translucent, perfect for all kinds of sex.

Red light bulbs in a couple of your bedroom lamps and low lighting not only set a mood, but it also makes a declaration of sexual expectations. Ladies, you can create a signal to communicate your sexual intentionality to your partner in a novel way using those same red light bulbs. Then get into the shower to prepare yourself for the full sexual experience, including oral sex by washing with fresh-smelling feminine wash.

Preparing Your Body

Manicure, pedicure, and more—When a woman is anticipating a hot time in bed, this is just the time to head to the salon and get the full treatment, including pedicure, manicure, and perhaps an eyebrow threading or hair coloring.

Maybe even a bikini wax job to make your pussy sleek and inviting. Or maybe you'd like a Brazilian wax for total banishment of all pubic hair. Men have two main schools of thought about waxing and shaving the lady's pubic area. One, clean-shaven; two, naturally hairy.

One man explained to me that the pussy scent lingers in the hair that covers it. That seems reasonable, especially if you are enthralled with natural pussy odor. These cleave perfectly with the categories above.

If a man you are seeing prefers shaved pussy, and you are willing to offer that to him, you will need to add sufficient time to your emoluments and make sure that the implement you are using won't cause shaving nicks that are common with some cheap razors. I use one that is specifically designed for shaving intimate areas. The entire shaving area of the multiblade razor is surrounded with smooth and sleek and wide plastic edges and it works well.

Hair and bodily cleanliness—Need I remind the reader that I am a huge proponent of washing well before sex. This will ensure that the pussy is fresh and clean-smelling to the nose as well as the mouth, mainly in preparation for oral sex. One idea that I'll pass along is to wash your mouth out with hydrogen peroxide, the kind that comes in the brown plastic bottles, which minimizes germs and is tasteless. Of course you spit it out after swooshing it around in your mouth for no more than about ninety seconds, swish it through the teeth, and recommend a good rinse with warm water and maybe some extra brushing, or your tongue will look coated. Then brush teeth and tongue with a small amount of toothpaste and rinse again.

Ladies with dentures, if you plan to perform fellatio (oral sex with your male partner), to prevent a mishap, you'd best secure your dentures or partials with denture adhesive.

Gentlemen, if you perform oral sex, you'd better secure your loose dentures or partials too.

Hydrogen peroxide is wonderful when used against a sore throat or gum inflammation, and gargling is a perfect delivery method because it helps your body fight off bacterial infections that often cause sore throats and inflammation. **It is important that you understand that you cannot swallow hydrogen peroxide under any circumstances.**

Hygiene is a huge factor, yet even more important is the assurance (or proof?) that your partner has been tested recently and is free of STDs (sexually transmitted diseases) and HIV/AIDS. Sometimes couples go together to be tested before having sex.

Rule 8: Cleanliness is essential, especially down there.

Pussy Smell: Natural or Carefully Washed

Female parts are complex, delicate, and subject to all kinds of issues, so it's important to pay close attention to important tips for personal care. I have always had a thing about being perfectly washed down there before sex. But I don't normally douche (wash out my vagina with a commercially available washing preparation or even just a quart of water) because the vagina's moisture makes it self-cleaning and has its own healthy balance. Of course, there are times that a nice warm douche is a must for your to-do list. Like when you just finished your period or recovered from a UTI or a fungal infection. I'm not going to go into the area of pussy-odor lovers, except to say they

202

are acknowledged to exist and to clarify, they don't prefer to smell a spanking clean pussy. They love to sniff dirty panties and fun things like that. Enough said. For some reason, I would have thought that a normal red-blooded American guy more often appreciates a pussy that's nice and clean. But no. Not always. Go figure.

According to the US Department of Health and Human Services' Office on Women's Health, in the United States, almost one in five women, fifteen to forty-four years old, douche regularly. Nevertheless, doctors recommend that you do not douche. Apparently douching can lead to health problems, including problems getting pregnant. Douching is also linked to vaginal infections and sexually transmitted infections (STIs).[1]

Pussy Soap

In addition to regular liquid or solid soaps of all kinds, I use a couple of different brands of special pussy-washing soap called feminine wash. These soaps are designed to wash but not impart perfumed odors or cause irritation. It is a special type of feminine wash. It is dye and scent free. Actually this product smells very fresh. One comes from a big retailer and costs around $2.75 for thirteen ounces. It produces a nice abundance of suds during the washing process and leaves you smelling fresher than newly mowed grass. All right, that is probably an exaggeration, but I'm sure you've got the picture.

Before Sex

This kind of natural smelling soap is highly recommended before sex, especially oral sex because it doesn't smell like something else, and it allows your natural smell to enhance the oral sex experience.

Note: The natural pussy taste and smell, unaided by any special fragrance, is very desirable to many people who

---

[1] Allaboutwomenmd.com.

eschew the artificial scents designed to cover up normal body odors. I call the kind of man who enjoys a natural pussy smell, "earthy."

Clearly this topic requires communication/conversation. An important one for people seeking a partner.

Men's Products

I vote for everyone—men and women—using the unscented fragrance-free washing products that are available on the market. If you already use a specific fragrance in a men's bodywash, cologne, or aftershave, you're excused, as long as you don't drown out your partner's fragrance in the process. If you are hesitant about wearing a strong aftershave or cologne, make sure it is a fragrance that she loves as much as you do. Aftershave closes pores, which makes the skin feel smoother and tighter. The fragrance of aftershave is less intense than cologne, so you may prefer to use it for that reason. Because of its skin-tightening properties, and the higher alcohol content, you should probably restrict aftershave to the areas of the skin and neck that are exposed to actual shaving because that is what it's designed to do.

Another uniquely masculine product is special antiperspirant that is formulated specifically for men, with stronger ingredients to deal with men's stronger odor.

Choosing a Fragrance

Of course, it's also your prerogative to wash with anything, including fragrant cherry soap if you want. I just prefer the smell to be clean to be able to experience the actual smell of the more natural secretions *down there* during oral sex after bath time. But I do normally use spray eau de toilette of whatever scent I'm wearing. That's the smell that I want him to find all over me, except places where you would like him to taste with his tongue. He doesn't want to dive in for some female scent and come up with a perfumy one instead. Avoid this when spraying scent all over you by shielding your pussy and nipples. Oh, and don't be stingy with the yummy scent. Just avoid spraying it directly on sexual parts of your body that may come into play with his/her mouth.

What scents to choose for a woman? I'm sure you've got your favorites, but in case you need a little assist, expensive musky scents are often the best. The floral Chanel 5 is always appropriate. Fragrance X offers their favorite scents for romance: spicy, floral, vanilla, musk, and lavender. This is a wide range of scents, and you are sure to find something perfect. If you fall in love with one of these scents, and if he really likes it, you might choose to make it your personal trademark and wear it every time you have sexual relations.

Making Sense about Scents

There is a triumvirate in the world of scents, and it plays out this way: eau de toilette and cologne versus perfume. According to Fragrance X, "the difference is simply the amount or concentration of oils in the fragrance. Eau de perfume has a higher concentration than eau de toilette, making it a stronger fragrance. There is also pure perfume, which has the highest concentration, and eau de cologne, which has the lowest concentration of oils." Aftershave comes last because it also contains ingredients that treat shaving cuts and nicks without excessive alcohol.

Rules about Scents

While I highly recommend that bodywash designed for the genitalia be neutral without fragrance, I am also a proponent of fresh-smelling floral bodywash for the entire body (except the genitalia). That said, I am also not big on fruit flavors of any kind and don't generally like heavily unctuous flowery scented fragrance. That leaves a huge field from which to choose. And if you are even slightly less selective than I am, a whole world of scents awaits you.

CHAPTER 33
WOMEN'S BODY HAIR
REMOVAL OR NOT

There are two major opposing schools of thought about women's body hair.

- **Pro: Shaving, waxing or depilatory, perfectly smooth**
- **Con: Removal (most or all body hair being retained)**

There are also variations that suit the individual.

Female Genital Area

There are ways to shave your pussy so that some hair remains but is neater than the natural pubic area bush. Or you can use a special razor for pubic area shaving that minimizes chances of nicks and cuts and shaves very close. Many salons offer service to remove most, if not all, pubic area hair with wax, and believe me, it is something that is better done by the professionals. Laser hair removal is also becoming more common.

Chemical hair removers—Chemical hair removers are not recommended for use on or near genitals. They are not, however, prohibited for the rest of the body, of course being subject to potential allergies or sensitivities. Test the product on a small area of your body to ensure that this doesn't happen.

Men's Body Hair and Beards

Despite the proliferation of short beards and bald heads, it seems that more men every day are getting into body hair removal, including back hair (thank God), chest hair, and pubic area hair. I'm going to theorize that men like to do it because it makes their *package* more prominent (larger) looking. No, let's face it; it's true that many men who *manscape* their pubic hair love the effect that it has on the perceived size of their penis, which seems larger because it's not hiding in a bush of hair. I believe that they have a point and find myself actually preferring *manscaped packages*. But I hate stubble with a passion. So there's that to contend with.

Challenge: Some men have a healthy growth of hair on both their penis and their testicles. Mainly because that hair grows back after shaving, causing stubble, this is not a desirable situation to most people, especially those interested in giving oral sex to their partner.

Solution: Daily shaving is necessary. So just accept it and do it if you always want to be as alluring as you can be.

More about Manscaping versus Shaving

The best way to manscape initially is with electric razor set at the height that cuts the hair to the length that you wish. This means that while shaving, you still leave at least a bit of fuzz behind. A clean shave means that there will be a prickly beard within twelve hours. That is why shaving is such an ordeal every single day. But some choose that daily effort because of the smooth baby skin left behind. Others keep a sharp and stylish beard that is soft enough not to cause irritation on the delicate skin of the genitalia. Sometimes the feeling of the beard on the skin is both erotic and exciting since the beard can be full of pussy scent after a session of oral sex. Sometimes the bearded one will decline to shower after sex just so he can enjoy smelling her pussy in his beard. It's very erotic, especially to those who respond to any perception of pleasure by all of the senses.

Tips for Shaving Pubic Hair

Gillette, the old standby shaving cream, razor, and blade company, offers a webpage called Tips for Shaving Pubic Hair.[1] This page is directed at men. There is also a selection of webpages with manscaping tips with the Gillette electric styler. They will undoubtedly interest and educate any uninitiated men about the comparatively new world of manscaping.

Waxing and Chemical Hair Removers

The waxing world of hair removal and its clients have been welcoming the recent phenomenon called Brazilian wax, which goes beyond other methods of waxing in that it offers complete pubic hair removal, from the front of the pubic bone to the area underneath, called the perineum, to the anus.[2] And then, there are the adherents of the depilatory method of chemical hair removers in which the product is spread on the areas of skin where hair is customarily removed with care around areas of sensitive skin. These products are spread over hairy areas, left on for about four minutes, and then rinsed off in the shower as they chemically dissolve the hair.

---

[1] https://gillette.com/en-us/shaving-tips/manscaping/pubic-hair-shaving.
[2] https://www.healthline.com/health/beauty-skin-care/what-is-a-brazilian-wax# brazilian-vs-bikini.

CHAPTER 34
OTHER PHYSICAL EXTRAS TO ENHANCE YOUR ENCOUNTERS

Eyelashes

Author Ashley Fetters wrote an article for the CUT called "What is the Point of Long Eyelashes?"

> Eyelashes are one of the few types of female body hair to make it into the "good, emphasize" category and not the "bad, eliminate" one...the pervasive notion remains that thick, soft lashes are for the ladies.[1]

Notes about Tattoos and Piercings

The arts of tattoo and piercing have grown exponentially in the past few years. You could probably say that the ancient arts of tattoo and piercing are experiencing a revival. An article about this growing phenomenon is found at Psychologized.org, called the "Psychology

---

[1]   https://www.thecut.com/2018/04/the-psychology-behind-why-we-like-long-dark-eyelashes.html.

of Tattoos, Body Piercings and Sexual Activity." Interestingly it points out that "people with tattoos thought themselves to be more sexy with it and 21% said that they feel more attractive and strong." It also points out that "the most popular body modification in the U.S. is ear piercings at 49% but having a body piercing on another part of the body is far less popular at only 7%."[2]

If you want to be literally blown away by the variations of piercings possible on the human ear alone, just visit Google with a couple of obvious search words like *pierced ears*. The photography that results is awesome, indeed.

Tattooed (Permanent) Makeup

Tattooed makeup has been in vogue for quite some time now. The tattooed makeup is used commonly for eyeliner, eyebrow accentuation, and lip liner. *Huffington Post* featured an article online called "Everything You Need to Know Before Getting Tattooed Eyeliner."[3]

More about Piercings: Tongue Piercing

If you enter "pierced tongue" into the Google search engine, you will be deluged with what seems like hundreds of photographs of pierced tongues that appear in the results. Other categories of information in the results include "healing," "infected," "swollen," and "pain" warn ahead of time of difficulties inherent in piercing the tongue. If you choose to do it anyway, there is online information about stimulating your partner sexually with your piercing. Now aren't you just dying to get your tongue pierced? Seriously now, piercings and tattoos have been around for thousands of years. They aren't going away anytime soon.

---

[2] https://www.psychologized.org/psychology-of-tattoos-body-piercings-and-sexual-activity/.
[3] https://www.huffpost.com/entry/what-to-know-tattooed-eyeliner_n_5b1fcc00 e4b0adfb826ded37.

A website called She Knows features an article entitled "The Sex Pros and Cons of Piercing," by Ashtyn Evans, that points out that the most common part pierced for sexual pleasure is the tongue. Evidently the positioning of the studs on the surface of the tongue gives pleasure to both the penis and the vulva/clitoris. "When used for oral sex, the small metal ball or tongue ring that is on the tip of the ring will add pressure, tease, and bring a new sensation to the experience for your lover. People who use them seem to get off on the fact that their partner enjoys oral sex so much."

Cosmopolitan Magazine's "14 Things to Know Before Getting a Tongue Piercing"4 is interesting for obvious reasons, but it is a very practical guide to doing it correctly while minimizing potential for issues to arise.

Nipples

I think that the medical community already established this as fact, but in my opinion, breasts and nipples are both part of a major sexual system. Nipples and breasts are not only part of the reproduction system, they are also part of the sexual process that leads to it, if you get my logic.

Although it's less common for men, both men and women commonly experience nipple stimulation during sex, which doubles the reason for their inclusion in the conversation that you have with each other before going to bed for the first time together. One time, I had sex with a man whose nipples were so sensitive that when I touched them lightly, he immediately had his orgasm. Clearly he should have told me. It was an abrupt ending to a very hot session.

Nipple Piercing

The subtitle to a *Cosmopolitan Magazine* article, entitled "Nipple piercing pain and benefit, and everything you need to know… They can

---

4   https://www.cosmopolitan.com/sex-love/a10392687/tongue-piercing-faq/.

feel amazing when touched during sex." I don't know about you, but that statement makes me want to know more.

Nipple Orgasms? Who Knew?

Some people say when their pierced nipples are flicked, licked, or massaged, it really adds to their arousal. In fact, nipple play alone can end in an intense orgasm (yes, nipple orgasms exist), and this is supposedly more likely to happen if you have them pierced.[5]

Genital Piercing (Female)

Genital piercing is a form of body piercing that involves a part of the genitalia, thus creating a suitable place for wearing jewelry… In, addition, some piercings enhance sexual pleasure by increasing stimulation. (for both the wearer and partner) Genital piercings can be found in many tribal societies, in particular in South and East Asia, where it has been part of traditional practice since ancient times. Early records of genital piercing are found in the Kama Sutra over 2000 years ago.[6]

Female genital piercings that are reported to enhance pleasure are the piercings that pass through or close to the clitoris, i.e. the clitoris piercing and the clitoral hood piercing.[7]

---

[5] https://www.cosmopolitan.com/uk/love-sex/sex/a9609890/nipple-piercing-pain-facts/.

[6] https://en.wikipedia.org/wiki/Genital_piercing.

[7] Ibid.

Due to genital physiology, women seem to gain more sexual pleasure from both, their own as well as her partner's genital piercings.[8]

Genital Piercing (Male)

Additionally genital piercings can enhance sexual pleasure during masturbation, foreplay, and intercourse. While female genital piercings do this only to the women wearing them, male genital piercings can enhance stimulation for both the person wearing the jewelry and their partner by stimulating both the glans of the wearer and the vaginal wall or the anus of the penetrated partner. Due to genital physiology, women seem to gain more sexual pleasure from both, their own as well as her partner's genital piercings. Possible piercing sites on the male genitalia include the glans, the skin of the penis shaft, the scrotum, or the perineum.

---

[8] Ibid.

CHAPTER 35
SEXUALLY STIMULATING GETUPS

Although heterosexual men generally don't dress up for sex, their partners often will, and depending on the sex they are planning to have, one of them may or may not change their mind and ultimately decide to dress up for sex. Whether that means role-play outfits, sexual fantasy costumes, leather, lingerie, or hard-core *B and D, S and M*—all depends on your mood and how you decide to set the scene. You may even go for the idea of cosplay, the purpose of which is to dress up in a costume depicting your favorite character in fiction, nonfiction, or the movies. There are variations on the theme as well. Check out this article online, "Cosplay 101: Everything You Need to Know About It," by Rhys McKay.[1]

Feminine Clothing

Clothing that is regarded as feminine ranges from innocent lacy nighties to how about a lacy black teddy with black thong, black garter belt and stockings, and two-inch black heels on up to feminine

---

[1] https://certifiedcomic.shop/blog/cosplay-101-a-beginners-guide-to-cosplaying/.

role-playing costumes. Oh, by the way, a naked woman is feminine too, but some women are self-conscious and need a little nudge.

Provocative Makeup for Women

Makeup starts with foundation, including over the neck and down to top of breasts. Complete with highlighter blended down the center of the face, blush on cheeks, and eyelids topped with black eyeliner, eye shadow, and deep-colored, especially red, no-smear lipstick.

What's Hot and Masculine

Men don't need to do much to look like men, except a touch or two that's suggestive at a very elemental animal level. Shirt, open at the neck, reveals a slightly hairy chest. Warm. Skin-tight jeans has a great body inside. Hot. Wearing only a thong with the family jewels nestled in a fold of fabric. Hotter. Naked with a hard-on. Hottest.

Mirrors

Mirrors are HOT. One wall of my master bedroom is entirely mirrored with copious storage inside with all kinds of sexy stimulation outside for the very visual man, who likes to gaze at the mirror to watch himself. If you don't have any mirrors in your bedroom, consider installing one on the ceiling above your bed for the ultimate visual entertainment. Did I say mirrors are hot?

Do Alcohol and Drugs Enhance or Detract?

Even if we don't engage in it ourselves, we've all heard about people using certain alcoholic drinks, various pharmaceuticals, medical marijuana, and street drugs to enhance their sexual experiences. Derived from marijuana, CBD oil helps in the production of serotonin and dopamine, both of which ease depression and make the user more energetic.

Note from author: For the purposes of this book about developing healthy sexual relationships, I've decided to steer clear of discussing alcohol and drugs at all, except to say that excess alcohol is a known deflator of the hard-on, can literally destroy lives and kill you and your loved ones. As can many drugs. Enough said.

Wineglasses

When I serve guests any beverage, I like to use extra-large wineglasses. It just seems more festive that way. And for those who don't imbibe alcohol, I love to serve juice concentrates diluted with filtered water. I usually stock pomegranate, blueberry, tart cherry, and cranberry juice, which can be diluted with club soda instead. I call them fruit coolers, and they are very delicious and refreshing, both during and after sexual marathons.

CHAPTER 36
SENSUAL FOODS

The important place that food occupies in the sexual/romantic setting cannot be overemphasized. If you don't understand this, watch the movie *Tom Jones* with your significant other. Pay special attention to the famous eating scene in which they seduce each other with their eyes as they hungrily rip food off the bone with their teeth like cavemen after the big hunt. All I can say is apply knowledge gained. Food can taste so good and be so enjoyable to eat when you are turned on. Or you might find yourselves using food items to play with in bed. It can also be enjoyed for an après sex picnic in bed.

The Best Timing for a Romantic Dinner

The time will come when you realize that you cannot avoid the romantic dinner any longer (note: if you are incompetent in the kitchen, you must foot the bill at a restaurant). If you are reasonably competent in the kitchen, you should plan to prepare anything with wine; if not, use concentrated soups as ingredients in a chicken dish with fresh sautéed mushroom slices, dry white wine, and a can of cream of mushroom soup. Don't forget to add your cooked chicken breasts. Serve with pasta to soak up that sauce. Enough recipe-making. This is a sex book, not a cookbook.

Best Presex Food

I don't think I need to point out that you should eat light before engaging in sex. With that said, I can certainly suggest foods that would not overpower but actually help to fuel your activities. You might select clean, raw, and fresh food like vegetable crudités, carrots, celery, broccoli, cauliflower, cherry tomatoes, as well as protein in the form of thin-sliced ham and roast beef, thin-sliced mild cheese, perhaps some cashew nuts and fresh fruit like grapes. That should do it.

Best Food for Sex Play

This is a true story, I swear. There was a time, not too many years ago, that I took up with long cucumbers. It's true. For some crazy reason, I wanted the long kind of cucumbers to put up inside my vagina which have a long "handle." God's honest truth. I bet you've never seen that anywhere—sex with a cucumber carefully washed and allowed to come to room temperature before use. The embarrassing thing that I used to do when I bought packages of fresh cucumbers, I'd show the package to the gal working the self-service registers and whisper in her ear, "These are the best dildos." And then I'd wait for her response (it was always an embarrassed laugh). I'm so naughty.

Food Fit for a King and Queen

Cold lobster meat just out of the shell, cold shrimp, oysters on the half shell, rolls of sliced, rare roast beef, freshly cooked artichoke hearts with melted butter and lemon juice, and more. Great for après sex hunger.

Types of Suitable Foods for a Sex Picnic in Bed

My idea of fun food to eat in bed might include cold chicken (on the bone or not), cold shrimp cocktail, sushi (mainly rolls), sliced mangoes, peaches (in season), cantaloupe, your favorite nuts and dried fruit, and anything else that strikes your fancy. Of course, you could always serve oysters Rockefeller and strawberries dipped in chocolate. It's up to you.

CHAPTER 37
SEXUAL LUBRICANTS

Sexual lubricants should probably go without saying. I mean, if you use it, everything is easier. When her vaginal lubricant runs dry—which it eventually does—I'm a great proponent of using virgin coconut oil.

Coconut Oil (Heated Up)

Coconut oil (natural virgin) comes in fifty-two-ounce containers which I keep in my kitchen to heat up in the microwave for a minute before using for massage or sex. I had used it recently with anal sex, and it performed wonderfully. I highly recommend the use of coconut oil, which is good for skin and scalp as well as cooking. Healthline.com put together an informative piece on the issues about coconut oil that are worth reading, for safety's sake.

Commercial Lubes

There is no substitute for a visit to the sex store to locate other commercial lubes. I can only say that AstroGlide, Kama Sutra Oil, and KY Jelly are three other lubricant products that I have used in the past and enjoyed for various reasons. Each is different. But please note that despite being a superior product, Kama Sutra is virtually impossible to get these days. KY Jelly is an old standby. It's important to have at least one lube product in the top drawer of the nightstand at all times.

Author Reveal

When I had a rich stockbroker boyfriend many years ago in New York, he used to come over and bring a catered steak dinner from one of the fancy steak houses in the city. He was really good to me and had a great imagination, especially about places to entertain his friends. One time he rented the first floor of a town house in the city for a party. There was a sauna and a swimming pool, and quickly it became a mostly nude sexy event for everyone. And one of my first girl-on-girl sexual experiences, the first in front of the partygoers. Talk about showing off.

Another time, he rented a small RV and dressed his friend up as a chauffeur and off they went around Manhattan, parking and calling his friends from a phone booth on the street at lunchtime. As I arrived downstairs from my office, I was immediately escorted into the RV and offered a glass of champagne and a sandwich. There was definitely some sex too. Those were the good old days, years ago, in New York.

CHAPTER 38
SEX TOYS

I finally took my own advice and went to the website of the major online sex toys purveyor. And I learned a few things I didn't know about sex toys.

Dildos

First there are the suction-cup dildos. I'm not too clear about where you're supposed to mount them in order to mount them yourself. All I can think of is the front of the refrigerator. In theory, these suction-cup things are good because they free up your hands to do other things. Like what? I'm confused. But wait. It also has something to do with strap-on harnesses for simulated penis-to-vagina sex between women, also called strap-ons. There's also pegging, a role-reversal with the woman strapping on the dildo and fucking her male partner's ass. That's an evocative visual, isn't it? I love it.

Dildos range from realistic dildos to vibrating dildos, huge dildos, glass dildos, anal dildos, G-spot dildos, double dildos, black dildos, and thirty-seven different strap-ons.

Vibrators

This is where you'll find your seven-inch vibrator, your eight and ten-inch whoppers, some with, some without testicles. You'll also find rabbit vibrators, clit vibrators, wand massagers, bullet vibrators, G-spot vibrators, realistic vibrators, anal vibrators, classic vibrators, luxury vibrators, and finger vibrators. Phew. I'm exhausted.

I just had to know how the rabbit vibrators work. It provides clitoral stimulation at the same time as it provides penetration. I have several vibrators on my shopping list to find out exactly how the newfangled ones work. Bullet and finger vibrators. Hmm.

While exploring the world of vibrators, I came across the Power Pounder Thrusting Dildo and the Gyrating Ass Thruster. Don't you just love the names they give these things? Creative and evocative. The same site has the "Ultimate Vibrators Guide," "10 Best Vibrators Ranked & Reviewed," "Vibrators 101: Beginning Guides, Rabbit Vibrator Guides, Wand Massager Guides."[1]

Butt Plugs

I'm ridiculously new to the world of butt plugs, which are perfect for training a person's anus to open more readily for anal sex. Butt plugs often come in three sizes. Need I say small, medium, and large? Anyone can play with them for the erotic effect they give. Male, female, straight, gay, and everything in between.

But wait. There's more. Under butt plugs, one website offers prostate toys, anal beads, trainer kits, anal dildos, lubes, and douches. And not only are these products sorted by price, you can compare size, material, color, rating, features, and still more. The world of sexual accessories goes on and on. Another result of that same search quickly yielded another with fox tails of various colors attached to butt plugs. Does the creativity in the sex toy world seem to go on and on? Yes. And that's the whole idea—not to take ourselves so seriously. Just have fun and be responsible to your partner.

---

[1] Visit Adam & Eve.com vibrators for practical information about how to use a rabbit vibrator.

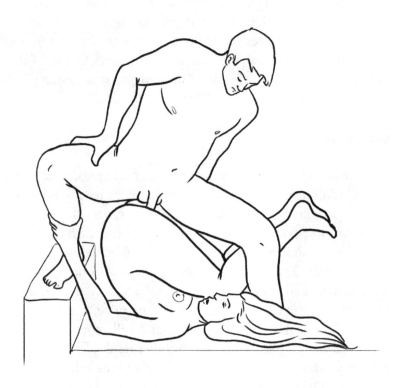

Lubes and Lotions

I keep reading that water-based lubricants are the ones to use during sex because the condom will remain intact. But finally I found the facts on a Healthline page about water-based lubes; it seems that water-based lubes can be used in practically any activity you can think up, even ones involving silicone toys. Water-based lubes are also safe to use with condoms.[2]

An anal sex product that might be crying out to be used? Desensitizing gel. Silicone-based sex lube is extra slippery for lasting sex sessions. The largest site for toys and lubes (adameve.com) offers male sexual enhancers, bath and body products, anal lubes, flavored lubes, massage oils, female sexual enhancers, silicone lubes, and hybrid lubes.

Massage

There's nothing like a full body massage and scalp treatment with warm coconut oil, but you may decide to stop greasing each other up to the point that you will surely slip if you both lie down together. You need a little friction to have sex.

Note: If slipping around with your partner is your idea of fun, all you need to do to protect your bed from the mess is put down a large shower curtain covered with a fitted sheet, go ahead and have a slippery time of it. Just don't slip on your way to the shower.

> **Important note about *autoerotic asphyxiation* (AEA):** Because I like to wear ribbons quite tightly wrapped around my throat, I've made allusions to AEA in the past, as if it was just something novel, interesting, but after research and learning about accidental deaths during masturbation, I decided to steer clear of it here.

---

[2] "Lube Shopping Guide," Healthline.

Happy Ending

At the end of a conventional massage, it's wonderful to have what is called "the happy ending," which might consist of oil infused masturbation and oral sex. Maybe even sex. Break out the massage table. Oh, on second thought, I'm not entirely sure that two should try to have sex on a massage table. It probably isn't sturdy enough for two.

Edging

Edging is the thing at present. People are talking about it. Yet quite a number of people, including men, have never heard of it and don't know how it works. Many haven't tried it yet. Now that may have been the case several years back, but I've become aware of it, especially lately when talking to a hot man. The hottest men have already done it. The hot man is definitely interested in it. The shy man who knows nothing about edging will have his ever-loving mind blown when he is edged for the first time.

Here is the description of an edging session. The man is lying on the massage table, cock-side up. Coconut oil is warm and in a bowl nearby. Soft sexy music is playing in the background. The woman performing the edging wears very little clothing for easy access during the massage table edging session. She takes her first warm coconut oil and gently handles his cock and balls to coat them with the oil. She masturbates him for a while until he starts to get hard (of course, if he is already hard, she will work with that too, the best she can).

She bends down and takes his cock in her mouth and slowly starts to suck him. Moments later, when he's becoming excited, she stops all stimulation. She stands completely still, holding his cock and balls in each hand but completely still. A few long moments later, she resumes contact and deep-throats him. She sucks his balls gently and goes back to deep-throat again. She stops completely. He squirms with desire for more. He'll be ready to cum soon, but not so fast, she says. Next she masturbates him slowly once again, then a bit

226

faster and more deliberately. And the cycle goes on until forty minutes have passed. By this time, he is beside himself, wanting to cum, and she is trying valiantly to keep that from happening by taking him to the edge over and over again. It is truly exquisite torture that leads to a huge payoff at the end.

Hair-Pulling

During the heat of sex, usually fucking from behind in the doggy-style position, her hair becomes a great target for pulling, especially if it's long, which is common nowadays. It also helps when the hair is thick and plentiful because there's no fear of losing any of it if he gets out of control. I happen to enjoy it myself because I have long and thick hair, which is usually up in a ponytail and easy to grab from behind.

Spanking

Spanking is fun the same way hair-pulling is fun. It's a bit naughty, and keep in mind that the pressure exerted doesn't have to be too intense, and it should never be. You shouldn't leave red hand marks all over her days after a spanking. That happened to me once. The guy didn't know his own strength. After that time, when I admonished him, he was gentle as a lamb.

B and D

Now for a few words from the world of bondage and discipline, also known as B and D, a term that is defined by encyclopedia.com as:

> The consensual physical restraint of a sexual partner for the purpose of inflicting pain, punishment, or humiliation. Serious Bondage and Discipline, however, is practiced by a much narrower portion of the general population and

is commonly engaged in by men and women participating in sadomasochism and domination and submission activities."

I don't mean to sound dramatic, but that's the unvarnished truth.

CHAPTER 39
LIGHT BONDAGE
AND DISCIPLINE

The few times that I've been bound with rope don't stick out much in my memory, except one time, with a long chain of ugly neckties; I found it quite fun. One of my ankles was tethered to the doorknob, I remember. To me, the most logical way to bind anyone is spread-eagle, legs tied to the bottom legs of the bed and arms tied at the upper two legs. I do remember that that one really made me squirm. But that was enough. I really don't get off on being restricted in my movement. Each to his or her own.

Soft Rope

I've got several lengths of soft rope in my bedside table just in case the need arises. We shall see. Soft rope is better because it doesn't burn the skin like the rougher kind. I suppose if the idea of being bound with rope were more appealing to me, I'd have more to say, but this is all I have.

Foot Fetish

I'm getting a bit of a complex trying to compare my advanced sexual experience, and all I find is that I am a lightweight. I've had only one wannabe foot fetishist who got off on sucking my toes. I have to say that he did it so well that I actually enjoyed it. It's one of those sensations that is hard to forget once you've had the experience. A serious fetish is often a focus that demands to be acted out night and day.

> Toe kissing and sucking, watching videos of feet, taking photos of a partner's feet, rubbing someone's sweaty feet after a workout, genital stimulation with feet, or describing foot odor to one's partner are some ways a foot fetish can be played out, says Ashley Grinonneau-Denton PhD, certified sex therapist and co-director of the Ohio Center for Relationship & Sexual Health.[1]

Subtypes of foot fetishes exist, too, like this one. "Some people love to worship adorned feet, whether with jewels, tattoos, nail polish, feet in heels, socks, stockings, or bare feet," sex therapist Moushumi Ghose, owner and director of Los Angeles Sex Therapy, tells *Health*.[2]

Dominatrix

One of my very close friends (who will remain nameless) actually role-played a dominatrix on a regular basis for a while and found willing guys to be her submissive sex partners. I'm not sure how long this went on—probably no more than a year or two—but I remember thinking that I could do that, if I wanted to. I just never wanted to. It has to do with control and lack of control. And I am told that I am not a control freak. Thank God. But for the person who loves having that sense of control, this is the ideal game to play—dominatrix and submissive.

---

[1] https://www.health.com/condition/sexual-health/foot-fetish.
[2] Ibid.

Submissive

It's probably no surprise to you that I finally identified to myself first, and the world second, I am a traditional female submissive. That does not mean that if I have an idea for the next sex play, that it isn't going to fly when I share it with him. Men are imaginative about sex, but sometimes they appreciate some creative suggestions here and there.

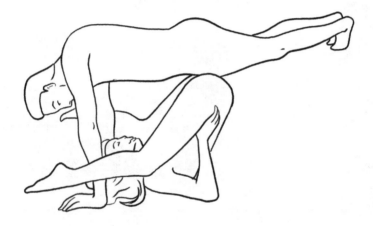

Fingers

During oral sex, I always enjoy at least one finger to be up inside me at some point, either my pussy or my anus. Given the fact that it's not a difficult task, it should be a regular occurrence in a great sex life. Fingers supply a rhythmic source of stroking to genitalia and nipples until reaching orgasm. If you are doing this for another person, ask first about preferences. Make sure hands are freshly washed. Avoid long nails. If nails are too long, use a dildo instead.

Fisting

Fisting is entirely different and a curiosity for a lot of people. And I wish I understood the attraction to fisting as a sexual act. It is mainly utilized by gay men and notoriously occurred at the Catacombs in San Francisco until the HIV scare of the 1980s.[3] For a ton of information about this, if you are curious, consult Google and go to Wikipedia for the complete story on fisting. Although DVDs are quickly becoming passé because of streaming content from such sites as Pornhub, you also should be able to get a DVD at the local sex shop that features fisting.

> Assignment 3: Go to a sex store and try to rent a DVD about fisting (if they still carry DVDs). Streaming video of that is probably also available online. The salespeople work in the sex store to help you. Don't feel embarrassed or self-conscious asking for direction. They can be of a huge help to you, and they are asked a thousand embarrassing questions (and of course, while there, see what else you can buy, such as lube, a vibrator for your partner, or perhaps a couple of role-play costumes).

---

[3] "Fisting," Wikipedia.

Anal Sex

According to Wikipedia entry about anal sex, the abundance of nerve endings in the anal region and rectum can make anal sex pleasurable for both men and women. That's not to say that everyone should experience it. It means that those who wish to engage in anal sex should be given that opportunity by accommodating partners. "Anal sex without protection of a condom is considered the riskiest form of sexual activity and therefore health authorities such as the World Health Organization (WHO) recommend safe sex practices for anal sex."

Occasionally I enjoy anal sex, and that's only been the case since I've been on the bioidentical hormones that make me horny as a herd of goats. No joke. Enough said.

CHAPTER 40
THE PENIS

It is my considered opinion that each man on this earth regards his penis as the center of the world—no, the universe. Even when a guy's cock is well under eight inches, he will send you online photos of it as if it were the largest most beautiful penis you'll ever see. What's important is that the man sporting that penis should be taking care of himself with proper diet and limited alcohol, and perhaps trying some supplements and herbs. There's also the possibility of getting testosterone via bioidentical hormones, or some guys prefer testosterone shots. Some of these items have the capacity to increase or decrease sexual response. There are different hormone products that should be explored thoroughly and in conjunction with medical professionals to provide direction.

Oh! I nearly forgot. So why does the conversation always boil down to the size of a guy's penis? Does it really matter? There are different schools of thought about that. One school is that bigger is better. But some women are not built for a large penis. And many of them are afraid of a large penis because of fears of choking during oral sex. That's good news for the guys with a smaller penis. And more good news, she can accommodate more of him in her mouth and toward the back of her throat when she performs oral sex. So in a number of ways, smaller actually ends up being preferable in some ways.

In my day, they always used to say, "It's not the size of your boat but the motion of the ocean." That seems purposefully vague to me. What do you think? *Science* magazine did a study back in 2015 about the average-size penis when flaccid and when erect. The results were surprising to me, and I'll tell you why. "The average flaccid, pendulous penis is 3.61 inches in length. The average erect penis is 5.16 inches long."[1] I never expected to learn these relatively unimpressive statistics, but more important is the fact that my previous impressions were so wrong, and now, I will change my expectations going forward. Better yet, don't judge penis size as if that knowledge is all you need about a man's ability to satisfy in a multitude of ways. When you learn more about this, you will realize that the male body offers so many ways to sexually express to you if you can just relax, be 100 percent in the moment, and enjoy yourself. If you are willing, he will transport you to your sexual bliss.

More about Penis Sizes: Bigger Than Normal

The few men with large penis sizes that I've been to bed with certainly stick out in my memory (sorry, bad pun). I have to admit it. That's not to say that those men were necessarily stellar in bed. Why? Because great sex isn't dependent upon size but other things like experience, energy, intensity, passion, gentleness, and more that haven't occurred to me yet. That may seem a bit sacrilegious to some who (mistakenly) believe that size is the most important factor.

> **Circumcision is the removal of the foreskin from the human penis. In the most common procedure, the foreskin is opened, adhesions are removed, and the foreskin is separated from the glans. After that, a circumcision device is used so the foreskin is uniformly cut off all the way around.**

---

[1] Sciencemagazine.org.

Circumcised or Natural Foreskin

The decision whether or not to have your baby boy circumcised is apparently under increasing consideration nowadays in the United States more than Europe, where the practice is not performed and, in fact, questioned. Religious Muslims generally have their baby boys circumcised, largely as a ritual, with the ultimate benefit being increased cleanliness. Jewish practice is for a circumcision ceremony with a rabbi, called a *bris,* which is attended by the community of close family associations/rabbi and family members generally on the eighth day of the baby boy's life.

An article in *Quartz,* January 17, 2017, online magazine, entitled "The industrialized world is turning against circumcision. It's time for the US to consider doing the same:"

> The medical community seems to disagree: both the U.S. Centers for Disease Control and Prevention (CDC) and the American Academy of Pediatrics (AAP) claim the benefits of circumcision outweigh the risks, citing evidence that circumcision lower a man's risk for HIV, urinary-tract infections and penile cancer. Neonatal circumcision has been the most common surgery in America for over a century. Today, nearly six out of ten newborns are released from hospitals foreskin-free.[2]

Oral Sex: Mind Over Matter

Oral sex is that elephant-in-the-room kind of subject that no one wants to be the one to bring up. I say bring it up, and do that early in the game. Ladies, if you are looking for a man who will go down on you as a regular thing (and not a token thirty seconds' worth), you will learn to steer clear of those who really don't do it.

---

[2] "Why is circumcision so popular in the US?" *Quartz,* qz.com.

It's a matter of natural selection of a person's sexual style. And there's nothing wrong with asking for what you need and want, especially since receiving (and giving) oral sex is a must on virtually everyone's list and the primary goal of this book. And your partner's oral skills may be lacking, so be patient as he/she perfects his/her technique.

Blow Jobs (Sucking Cock)

I just love the words that are used in these descriptive elements. Just understand, we never blow, we suck. And we certainly don't suck a cock. That would make the cock mad. We suck a penis, a hard penis or a soft penis if need be. We also suck dick. Sorry, couldn't resist playing a bit. Yes, we definitely suck cock.

Developing Oral Skills

If you are lucky and don't have a well-developed gag reflex, you can learn to entertain at least seven inches of an eight-inch cock of a normal width. By the word *entertain*, I mean suck, deep-throat, and stroke with your hand and tongue. Some people can get more of it down their throats. With practice, the level of comfort may improve to the point where the person doing the sucking actually craves to suck cock. Could that be the origin of the term *lucky stiff*?

Hand Job

A commonly applied foreplay technique, it is simple to give someone a hand job. Just grasp his penis and pump it slowly and deliberately. Have him show you what he likes, and do that over and over until he cums. Rinse and repeat (just kidding). He also might respond more quickly if you use warm coconut oil as a lubricant for your hand job. That's almost a guarantee.

A COMPLETE GUIDE TO PLEASURING YOUR PARTNER

To Swallow or Not, That's the Question

It's amazing how when you have that important conversation with a guy who is attracted to you, the question of whether you swallow ejaculate or not is always a key answer for him to get early in the game. I never thought it was a major thing to think about. Apparently I was wrong about that. I found an article entitled "What to know about swallowing semen" that immediately states that "although swallowing semen is a relatively safe and common practice, there are some risks to be aware of. However, the CDC explains that the risk of transmitting an STI such as HIV through oral sex is low."[3]

What to Look for in a Mate

This topic is the last in the book. I wanted to leave you with a bang. If a particular person is your sexual ideal, then there's a good chance that he/she would turn out to be a great mate when you aren't in bed together. Being highly attuned to each other sexually is actually enough for some couples to stay together with a fairly healthy bond. Others prefer the connection to be more spiritual. Still others look to get along with each other in day-to-day living for a deep long-term connection. It depends on what is most important to you. Just make sure you are operating from a place of selflessness, with positive communication and oral sex, of course!

---

[3] https://www.medicalnewstoday.com/articles/swallowing-semen#risks.

239

ACKNOWLEDGMENTS

Dineshkumar Viswanathan, for helping me to come up with the scope, concept, and theme of the book.

Brian Williamson Fisk, my younger brother, who egged me on to write the book already. David Collins Fisk was the (gay) middle child, who died of AIDS in 2001. We will never stop thinking of and missing that wonderful man.

Jeanine Gurian, my closest female friend who never lost faith in me.

NYU Film School, which helped to prepare me with their dramatic writing courses.

Dan Kleinman, my dramatic writing professor at NYU and who later taught at Columbia University Film School for twenty years.

Gregory Rodgers, my erstwhile husband, who has been there to encourage me and to help me along.

APPENDIX 1
IS PELLET HORMONE THERAPY FOR ME? WHAT YOU SHOULD KNOW ABOUT BIOEQUIVALENT HORMONES

WHAT ARE HORMONES AND WHY ARE THEY SO IMPORTANT?

In simplest terms, hormones are chemical messengers, produced by a group of glands known as the endocrine system that course through your bloodstream and enter tissues where they turn on switches to the genetic machinery that regulate everything from reproduction to emotions, general health, and well-being. Hormones can be thought of as the life-giving force that animates you physically, mentally, and emotionally. As hormone production decreases, the body often begins to slow down its rejuvenation and repair of tissues and organs. This can cause health to decline and aging to accelerate.

What Is Hormone Pellet Therapy?

Hormone pellet therapy is a state-of-the-art medical protocol, utilizing tiny hormone pellets that provide an on-demand delivery system to replenish the missing amounts of estrogen and testosterone. They are designed to supplement or add to your own hormones, not replace them. The pellets contain low-dose plant-based hormones derived from a naturally occurring compound found in soy and wild yam called diosgenim, which is biologically equivalent to human hormones. They are hand-formulated under sterile conditions in a licensing compounding pharmacy, using the purest ingredients and manufactured to the highest standards. The pellets are slightly larger than a piece of rice and are painlessly placed beneath the skin. Hormone pellet therapy allows your body to receive the balanced hormones it needs directly into the bloodstream, twenty-four hours a day, seven days a week.

Benefits include:

- Increased sex drive and satisfaction
- Increased energy levels
- Increased mental sharpness, concentration, and memory
- Improves sleep
- More stable moods; less irritability and grumpiness
- Decreased body fat
- Less anxiety and depression
- Increased sense of well-being
- Increased muscle mass and strength
- Increased bone density
- Reduced night sweats
- Reduced hot flashes
- Relief of migraines

How Long Has Pellet Therapy Been in Use?

Hormone therapy using pellets is not new. Hormone pellets were originally developed in France in 1935 to help alleviate the symptoms of menopause. They were first used in the United States from the early 1940s to the early 1970s, before synthetic hormones were heavily marketed, and are currently popular in Europe and Australia for both men and women.

What Are the Possible Side Effects?

There are very few side effects since the pellets are simply restoring the hormones to physiological levels. When first starting therapy, there will be a short adjustment period. The most common side effects are generally mild and can include temporary breast or nipple tenderness and temporary water weight gain.

How Do I Receive Treatment?

Make an appointment with a doctor with a practice in (Sottopelle) bioidentical hormone therapy. Together you will review your medical history and evaluate your symptoms. Lab studies will be measured to accurately determine your specified needs. Your treatment is based on your personal data and individual requirements. Next you will be scheduled for placement of the pellets which are inserted beneath your skin in the hip or buttock area. This is done in the office with local anesthesia and is similar to having an IV placed under your skin. This takes less than fifteen minutes, and once balance is reached, this needs to be performed twice per year.

How Safe Is It?

All estrogen is not the same. The estrogen that alarmed everyone is referred to as conjugated or synthetic. This (Premarin) is what was used in the study with unfavorable results. These hormones are botanical and are safer for you. As they are placed under your skin, they are directly absorbed and bypass the liver. This means that blood-clotting is not affected. In addition, there is no interference with medications taken for things like high blood pressure or heart disease. The botanicals do not increase the risk of breast cancer, and studies are ongoing which suggest that they are breast protective!

Dr. Philip Disaia (world-renowned cancer specialist) has even suggested that this form of estrogen be considered for patients with breast cancer. In studies, data has not revealed the estrogen to be a fuel to the fire when it comes to breast cancer. The debate further points out that risks of estrogen deprivation like osteoporosis do not bypass cancer patients. Dr. Gino Tutera (founder of Sottopelle) conducted a patient study (approximately one thousand patients over ten years) with a single case of breast cancer. The incidence of breast cancer in general is eight to nine cases per one hundred women.

APPENDIX 2
STATE AGE REQUIREMENTS (AGE OF CONSENT)

Table 1 State Age Requirements (Age of Consent)				
STATE	AGE OF CONSENT	MINIMUM AGE OF VICTIM	AGE DIFFERENCE BETWEEN THE VICTIM AND DEFENDANT (IF VICTIM IS ABOVE MINIMUM AGE)	MINIMUM AGE OF DEFENDANT IN ORDER TO PROSECUTE
Note: Some states have marital exemptions. This table assumes the two parties are not married to each other.				
Alabama	16	12	2	16
Alaska	16	NA	3	NA
Arizona	18	15	2 (defendant must be in high school and < 19)	NA
Arkansas	16	NA	3 (if victim is < 14)	20 (if victim is < 14)
California	18	18	NA	NA
Colorado	17	NA	4 (if victim is < 15), 10 (if victim is < 17)	NA
Connecticut	16	NA[11]	2	NA
Delaware	18[12]	16	NA	NA
District of Columbia	16	NA	4	NA

			Table 1	
		State Age Requirements (Age of Consent)		
STATE	AGE OF CONSENT	MINIMUM AGE OF VICTIM	AGE DIFFERENCE BETWEEN THE VICTIM AND DEFENDANT (IF VICTIM IS ABOVE MINIMUM AGE)	MINIMUM AGE OF DEFENDANT IN ORDER TO PROSECUTE
Florida	18	16	NA	24 (if victim is < 16)
Georgia	16	16	NA	NA
Hawaii	16	14	5	NA
Idaho	18[13]	18	NA	NA
Illinois	17	17	NA	NA
Indiana	16	14	NA	18 (if victim is > 14)
Iowa	16	14	4	NA
Kansas	16	16	NA	NA
Kentucky	16	16	NA	NA
Louisiana	17	13	3 (if victim is < 15), 2 (if victim is < 17)	NA
Maine	16	14[14]	5	NA
Maryland	16	NA	4	NA
Massachusetts	16	16	NA	NA
Michigan	16	16[15]	NA	NA
Minnesota	16	NA	3 (if victim is < 13), 2 (if victim is < 16)	NA
Mississippi	16	NA	2 (if victim is < 14), 3 (if victim is < 16)	NA
Missouri	17	14	NA	21 (if victim is < 14)
Montana	16	16[16]	NA	NA
Nebraska	16	16[17]	NA	19
Nevada	16	16	NA	18
New Hampshire	16	16	NA	NA
New Jersey	16	13[18]	4	NA

			Table 1	
		State Age	Requirements (Age of Consent)	
STATE	AGE OF CONSENT	MINIMUM AGE OF VICTIM	AGE DIFFERENCE BETWEEN THE VICTIM AND DEFENDANT (IF VICTIM IS ABOVE MINIMUM AGE)	MINIMUM AGE OF DEFENDANT IN ORDER TO PROSECUTE
New Mexico	16	13	4	18 (if victim is < 13)
New York	17	17	NA	NA
North Carolina	16	NA	4	12
North Dakota	18	15	NA	18 (if victim is < 15)
Ohio	16	13	NA	18 (if victim is < 13)
Oklahoma	16	14	NA	18 (if victim is < 14)
Oregon	18	15	3	NA
Pennsylvania	16	13	4	NA
Rhode Island	16	14	NA	18 (if victim is < 14)
South Carolina	16	14	Illegal if victim is 14–16, and defendant is older than victim	NA
South Dakota	16	10[19]	3	NA
Tennessee	18	13	4	NA
Texas	17	14	3	NA
Utah	18	16	10	NA
Vermont	16	16	NA	16
Virginia	18	15	NA	18 (if victim is < 15)
Washington	16	NA	2 (if victim is < 12), 3 (if victim is < 14), 4 (if victim is < 16)	NA
West Virginia	16	NA	4 (if victim is < 11)	16, 14 (if victim is < 11)
Wisconsin	18	18	NA	NA
Wyoming	16	N/A	4	NA

APPENDIX 3
QUIZ 1

Quiz 1: to take when halfway through *A Complete Guide to Pleasuring Your Partner: The Sex Education You Never Got.*

Terms for a woman's sexual organs.

1. Name of the outside of a woman's main sexual organ(s)
   a. Vulva   b. Vagina   c. Clitoris   d. G-spot
2. Name of the sexual organ that is at the center of a dynamite orgasm/outside and connects with another one inside—the G-spot.
   a. Vulva   b. Vagina   c. Clitoris   d. G-spot
3. Name of the passageway part of a woman's sexual organs. Babies are born through this passageway. It is where the man normally inserts his penis to have intercourse.
   a. Vulva   b. Vagina   c. Clitoris   d. G-spot
4. It's a small place inside a woman's anatomy that many people don't know that much about. For many people, it is a long journey to find it. It is located just inside at the top of the vaginal opening. It is accessed by fingers making a come-hither motion.
   a. Vulva   b. Vagina   c. Clitoris   d. G-Spot

Answers:

1. a
2. c
3. b
4. d

APPENDIX 4
QUIZ 2

Take this quiz when finished with *A Complete Guide to Pleasuring Your Partner: The Sex Education You Never Got.*

These address various terms for sexual preferences.

1. Term for women sexually/romantically preferring women.
    a. Lesbian   b. Gay
    c. Bisexual   d. Transgender
    e. Queer/Questioning
2. Term for an individual preferring men or women.
    a. Lesbian   b. Gay
    c. Bisexual   d. Transgender
    e. Queer/Questioning
3. Term for a person who has undergone sexual reassignment surgery to modify his/her sex organs to conform to the sexual preference he/she prefers. Note: there is a large segment of people who don't actually undergo the reassignment surgery but still consider themselves as part of that community.
    a. Lesbian   b. Gay
    c. Bisexual   d. Transgender
    e. Queer/Questioning

4. Term for homosexuals, either male or female.
   a. Lesbian   b. Gay
   c. Bisexual   d. Transgender
   e. Queer/Questioning

5. Term for an individual who is not settled into a gay lifestyle because he/she is not sure about being a full-blown
   homosexual.
   a. Lesbian   b. Gay
   c. Bisexual   d. Transgender
   e. Queer/Questioning

Answers:

   1. a
   2. c
   3. d
   4. b
   5. e

APPENDIX 5
A COUGAR AND
HER AMAZING CUB
Pamela H. Fisk

She uploaded five photographs of herself onto the best site for cougars and cubs. All of them full-length, no close-ups. One of them was quite revealing; she wore a white lacy robe that exposed an expanse of her breasts. The details of the photographs were good enough that it was clear she had no noticeable wrinkles on her face or neck. She clearly looked younger than her seventy years. And after some time passed, her experiences added up to a personal preference for cubs in their mid-to-late forties and fifties, but she had met a smattering of men in their sixties and early seventies who filled the bill very nicely when their time came.

That said, this particular cub is completely imaginary. Why? Because he's perfect, and no man is perfect. A gal can dream, can't she? So we will proceed. We'll call him Liam.

Liam's photograph and profile were the best she had seen on the cougar-cub site so far. He was the classically good-looking man. He was tall, dark, and handsome in a Yankee WASP way. Decidedly masculine. She decided that Liam was the man to pursue. Luckily she didn't have to suggest that he subsidize the expenses for his trip to see her. Clearly he was a man of substance.

She prepared for Liam's visit with the attention to detail that she was known for. She planned groceries for the picnic in bed that she planned. Shrimp. Sushi. Crudités. She gathered her clothes and lingerie. She bought fresh lilies to put in the bedroom and living room and roses to harvest the petals to spread on the bed. She set up hours' worth of sexy music. She brought out the battery-powered candles. She placed the fluffy fur on a corner of the bed, and when the time came, she would turn on a light that made the entire room glow in a hot and sexy coral color.

The personal preparations for the first night came next. She selected an outfit and laid it on the bed next to her dressing area. Then came her shower, which included a lot of shaving, careful pussy and butt-washing with special soap, in preparation for the oral sex that they would have during their sexual play together.

The bed was carefully protected against the fluid that her body would emit during the kind of sex you almost want to write home about. She carefully sprayed her body with the most delicious flowery eau de toilette that she had. She took care not to spray near her nipples or pussy.

Next came the one-piece black lace garter with black stockings attached. That was a struggle to get on right, but she was becoming an expert at it. Then came her black lace thong with a short string of pearls bridging her pussy from front to back. The demibra came next (it lifted her heavy DD breasts but didn't cover them).

Finally she put on the teddy lingerie that cupped her breasts in lace, covered her stomach, and revealed her rear, which was the perfect scene for him to see as he followed her into the apartment when he finally arrived. And of course, she put on sexy black faux suede boots, which never saw the light of day or a pavement outdoors but only her bedroom when she was feeling extra randy.

Next came the actual preparations since he was now only one and a half hours away. The bed was prepared. Shower. Shave. Completely clean with double-wash pussy and anus. Dressed. Makeup applied. A touch of exaggerated black on eyelids. Bright-red matte lip tint that is difficult to get off; a good thing. Great for kissing and oral sex. Hair pulled up in high ponytail, especially convenient for a little hair-pulling during sex from behind and amazingly effective as a youthful face-lifting style.

He came at the correct hour. They embraced and kissed. He felt her body against him. She explored his muscular back and ass as they stood there together in each other's arms. She offered him a drink, and he asked her what she had around. White wine. Red wine. Stella Artois. Presidente. A decent selection of hard liquor and Cognac. They walked together to the kitchen so she could serve him what he wanted. But he took over and handled drinks for both of them.

With drinks in hand, they sat together and talked. Their likes and dislikes. Their exercise programs. Their diet and sex life at present. They were having a lovely time together; this was their first date in a long time. Too long. At the end of their drinks, they both put down their empty glasses and embraced and soon were kissing each other hungrily. Perhaps easy to imagine, right then, the evening turned completely sexual.

He removed her hair fastener, and her thick hair immediately fell to softly frame her face. They gazed at each other hungrily. They didn't need to speak. She took his hand gently, and he responded to her touch sexually by becoming erect as she led him into the bedroom. They pulled off the bedding and put it aside for an exciting sexual interlude. He wanted to eat her pussy, and she was totally into that but wanted to suck him at the same time. Obvious solution—69, with him on top with his cock in her mouth under him for simultaneous stimulation and inevitable orgasm.

APPENDIX 6
BIG RED'S BJ

Anonymous

She was not a small lady. Didn't shop in the petite department. Although a little heavy, she was pleasing to look at and very sexy. I'm not going to tell you her name. I secretly called her Big Red. She had full nicely shaped pendulous breasts, with medium-sized light-brown nipples that she loved to have suckled. Her hair was reddish-brown, but she kept it dyed to a more striking red color so that men would notice her more. Not that they looked at her hair. She had large expressive bluish-green eyes and full pouty lips. To both of these features, she applied liberal amounts of makeup, accentuating them, adding to the attraction. She wore bras that pressed her breasts together, creating a canyon of cleavage, and tops cut low enough to make this effective. She "made eyes" at men everywhere she went. She would strike up intimate conversations with complete strangers and put her hands all over them, leaving whoever she was with looking foolish.

Her pussy hair was naturally bright red. She had a medium-thick bush that, even when freshly showered, retained her pungent alluring scent. She was always wet. I could reach into her pants at any random time, and her cunt would be thoroughly drenched, ready for action. Although there was some distance between us intellectually, I loved fucking her. She was so damned erotic. She was a passionate kisser. My dick felt great inside her. I would put her legs up on my shoulders and pound away on that pussy. She would grab me with the nails on both hands, dig in, and encourage me to ride her hard. The head of my cock often rammed up against her cervix. It was a sensation we could both feel, and we loved it.

I had lots of stamina, and she had lots of pussy to explore, so we enjoyed many long sessions that ended in fairly substantial orgasms for both of us. At the time, my dick could get hard again after cumming with about a twenty or thirty-minute break, so we had multiple sessions when we fucked over and over. One time we went on a weekend vacation. From Friday night to Sunday afternoon, we fucked twenty-seven times—no lie. Mostly all we did was fuck, eat, and doze during that trip.

Red was not afraid of the penis. When she wanted to fuck, she had no problem fondling my crotch, stroking my dick through my pants, pulling it out, playing with it, and other advances. She would readily go down on me. Her mouth was warm and inviting. She had sense enough not to be a biter. She could empathetically feel how well she was orally treating me and change up the action to meet my needs. But there was one problem. When fellatio got close to the point where ejaculation was likely to occur, she would remove her mouth and try substituting her hand. She acted like cum was a poison. She had good hand. But if you have good head going, and it gets switched up in the final few seconds, you're likely going to lose your edge. Many of you will be able to understand. If you're in a sexual situation that feels good, and you have an impending orgasm, and somehow that release gets interrupted, you're going to be left feeling cheated. I tried talking with her about it a few times, but she wasn't open to discussion. I would bring it up as we were engaging in foreplay. She would change the subject or get angry or start acting like her feelings were hurt, like she was being attacked. Anything but actual discussion.

Sexually that was our only real issue. I like my women to go down on me. I like the way it feels. I like to watch. I like to stroke her, to feel her pussy getting heated up while she's mouthing me. I don't always have to come in her mouth. Sometimes the urge takes me to just stop her, push her down on the bed, mount her pussy or ass, and fuck her like mad. So after several months of nongratification in fellatio, I knew I was going to have to get a handle on the issue.

One evening, we were getting heated up in foreplay, and it just felt like the right time to approach the subject again. We were naked. I held her close, and after breaking off a long kiss, asked her to look at me. She did but not in my eyes. I lifted her chin with my hand and looked her directly in the eyes. She had her hand on my prick. I asked her what she wanted to do with that and made it wag in her hand.

"I'll suck on it if you want," she said.

Still looking directly deep into the depths of her eyes, I said, "Yes, I'd like that. But only if you're going to really do it right. Otherwise I prefer that you not get me all excited, then let me down at the end."

She replied, "I've just always thought that was really yucky, so I've never tried it."

I replied, 'So how about trying it for me, and let's see how it goes?"

"Well, if you really want me to, I'll see if I can do it," she whispered.

We kissed a lot more. I was fondling and rolling her nipples around in my fingers and sucking them randomly. Sometimes I'd reach down and run a couple of fingers inside of her labia from bottom to top, gently brushing her clit. When I did this, she would breathe very heavily and arch her back, spreading her legs involuntarily. When there was a huge drop of precum at the tip of my cock, I reached down and smeared it on my fingertip, brought it up, and painted her lips with it. She sighed, and her body shook slightly. She looked at me lustily and took my turgid dick in a strong grip. She pursed her lips in a perfect round *O*, moved her head down, and put just the tiniest wet opening of her lips over the hole in my cock. Glancing up to ensure that I was watching her, she proceeded to slowly push the prick head into her firmly pressed-together lips. I started going nuts. The sensations were phenomenal.

She kept going, moving her hand, and sliding my dick in until she had my penis head in her throat and her lips buried in my pubic hair, something she had never done for me before. I was freaking fucking out. I realized then that she knew how to give a good blow job, but up till now, she had only been giving me the amateur version. She slowly slid my dick all the way back out of her mouth, keeping constant pressure on it all the way out to the tip. She got up, shifted around so she was between my legs, keeping constant contact between her mouth and my dick all the while. When she got settled comfortably, again the dick got sucked all the way into her throat, her lips nuzzling the base. Those big eyes were looking straight at me. I grinned widely and stroked her cheeks with the backs of my fingers. Slowly she lifted her mouth off me again. And went right back down on me. Up. Down. Up. Down. Constant pressure. When she went up, her tongue was circling the sensitive outer edge of my prick head. When her head was up, I could see how much saliva she had used to lubricate my fucker.

Now she tried some variation. One hand went down to cup my balls and gently manipulate them. With the other, she began adding fingers along with the upstroke of her head so that there was always a lot of contact on my prick. When she got to the point where she had her whole hand circling my cock on the upstroke, she began to variably move the hand from one side to the other or twist it while simultaneously pulling and maintaining a lot of suction. I was in fellatio heaven. I'd been with a couple of good dick-sucking women in the past, but now she had really stepped up. I tried to withhold my orgasm as long as possible in order to keep experiencing the pleasure, but I don't think I exceeded five minutes. She had me thrashing and bucking around like a mustang. She kept time right with all my reactions, determined to make this feel good for me.

There came a point where I could feel the precum leaking out of me continuously, like a line of fire running out of my balls through the head of my cock. It must have tasted good to her because she was making the same noises she made when she ate tasty food. I could tell by her actions that she was really getting into it, and I was glad because I was building up to a powerfully explosive orgasm.

She kept on, deep-throating me and fisting my prick, synchronized to my movements and reactions. I was losing the ability to think rationally. I felt one of her nipples brush my hand. I instinctively grasped it in my fingers and squeezed. She gasped, then increased the pressure of her mouth on my prick just a bit more. I was going completely wild now with all the stimulation.

On the next cycle of her going up and stroking her hand on me, I felt the head of my prick flare outward. All the sensitive little nerve cells around the edge were on fire. She immediately shoved her head back down on me, forcing my prick down her throat, and she grabbed my hips with both hands. At the same time, I felt an intense heat flash through my entire body. My heels and shoulders lifted, then banged down on the bed. My back stiffened. My hips splayed completely open flat, forcing my legs apart. My pelvis felt like it was trying to totally invert shape. My prick drove far, far down her throat, her eyes bulged and teared up a little. And the cum came pouring out of me like a fire hose. Involuntarily I yelled out, bucked, withdrawing my penis somewhat, and immediately rammed it back up into her throat. All the while, my balls were pumping and pumping load after load of cum into her face.

After the initial shock of how incredibly good it felt for her to do this for me, while I was still cumming, I looked down and watched her swallowing every pump of cum that shot out me. She was watching my reactions and was consequently reacting similarly to me. This was so damned hot that it just made me hornier than I already was. My cock stayed hard for an incredibly long time. She kept it in her mouth, licking, sucking, kissing, honestly making oral love to my dick, the way I'd been hoping she would for months. While doing this, she would occasionally glance at me and give me little smiles. Without words, I could tell that the experience had been just as enjoyable for her as it had been for me, and I was all warm and fuzzy inside.

When my cock finally couldn't take any more, and he shrank down a bit, she laid it gently on my leg, patted it, and sidled up to lie next to me, snuggling under my arm, her head on my shoulder. She looked up at me and, in a very tender voice, said, "Is that how you like it, honey?"

The palpable waves of passion flowing between our faces spoke more than mere words ever could, but I reassured her anyway by telling her that what she did for me was so much better than what I could have wanted her to do. I tried to lift myself from the bed, intending to make love to her but found my body almost incapable of movement. I was drained of energy, wrung out, almost unable even to think let alone act. She knew what I was trying to do and pushed me gently back down.

"You don't have to do anything," she said, "just relax and enjoy yourself."

I had no choice. There was no way I'd be able to do much. She laid her head down on my chest. I closed my eyes. One of the best sleeps of my life followed, without dreams or disturbances of any kind. From that time forward, she blew me in a similar way about once a week. I'm sure people could tell when I'd been given "the treatment" by the huge smile on my face.

APPENDIX 7
THE GAY PARADOX
Anonymous

What is the first thing we think of when we think of gay men? Queer eye for the straight guy? Gay men are supposed to have a gay gene that gives them a special fashion sense. Of course, it is not always true. Sadly I have many gay friends who have no fashion sense at all. Even so, we all know beauty when we see it. Our gaydar is always active and ever-focused on a cute smile, an amazing boy, or just some charming attitude. No matter how serious we may be in our professional lives, there is always a mischievous urge for a new conquest. Herein lies our dilemma. What is it we look for? What is it we really want?

It is funny how we ask people if they got lucky when they have a hookup. We have a fantasy that every sexual encounter is a memorable event, when the reality is far from it. A sexual encounter is kind of like a bullfight—there are a number of elements that have to come together for it to be a mutually satisfying experience. Both men must find each other attractive naked, but the human body can be deceptive when covered. There must be a mutual level of sexual stimulation. Nothing kills the experience as when one of the participants cannot get an erection or when he struggles to get his penis hard. And then there is the act itself. Too often it is a selfish conquest where one participant satisfies himself without any serious consideration of his partner's sexual gratification. Tops often forget to make sure the bottom is truly satisfied. It can also happen that one of the participants cannot reach orgasm. It is surprising how many gay men can only reach orgasm by themselves. I have a gay friend who told me he could never ejaculate with a partner.

There is a joke in the gay community. What is the definition of eternity? The answer is the time from when you come to when he leaves. Such is the nature of the hookup culture; a lustful quest for immediate gratification without repercussion or commitment. Many of us claim this is not who we are or what we want, yet it happens more often than we are willing to admit.

In my experience, there are two kinds of gay men: those who are in and stay in a relationship and those who don't. Many of my friends talk about the kind of person they want for a partner without ever finding Mr. Right. Obviously gay men are experts on relation-ships because they have had so many of them, yet the sad truth is that the qualities they look for are not the prerequisites of long-term partnerships. It is really quite paradoxical. They want the very thing they say they don't want. They don't want to be like their parents. They want to be free and spontaneous when long-term relationships endure because they are stable and predictable.

We often talk about the gay community when, in fact, it can be a very lonely place. If you ask me, the concept of community is aspirational; just wander through a gay bar on a Saturday night. We do make good friends, that is true. Who doesn't find their gay friends quite amusing? There is something about the gay gene that people love to tap into. There are so many gay men who are desperate to be needed and loved.

Doesn't gay mean happy? It has come to be an aspirational con-cept for most of us. Wander around in a gay bar (back when they were open), and you find a lot of sad and lonely men. It has been said that the average hookup occurs after just nine seconds, but after that, bar paralysis sets in. It would be curious to know what the average connection rate is. Chances are it is not that high. Most patrons go home alone.

Maybe we are just a superficial breed. We love pornography and images of hot men. A gay couple is pretty much an anachronism. We are, by nature, free spirits. A friend who had a tendency to be somewhat promiscuous would enjoy a date before opining, "He is not boyfriend material."

Yes, some of us do find long-term relationships, and some are actually monogamous, but they are the exception rather than the rule. For most, a relationship is more a period of transition than a happily ever after. People talk about starter houses and starter marriages. For most men, every relationship is a starter relationship, even if they last for decades. Even in the most committed couples, there is always conditionality. Circumstances can change everything, and so we live for the moment knowing that what is a loving and supportive relationship today may not be so tomorrow. That is the challenge, but achieving those moments of supportive love and affection is also the reward. It is an ephemeral reality we all live with.

Since generalizations are often wrong, it is impossible to generalize about gay attitudes and perspectives. Every coming-out story is different. Some are tragic and painful, while others represent a simple awakening. But what they do have in common, at a certain point, there is a realization of a sexual orientation. Whether and how it affects one's behavior can vary significantly. The fact is that the distinction between gay and straight is anything but clear-cut. Obviously some gay men only have sex with men, but many straight men pursue sexual encounters with men. There are many go-go bars across the country where many of the dancers will tell you they are straight.

So what does it really mean to be gay? Is it just a preference for the pole versus the hole? Clearly not, and this may be the ultimate paradox: being gay is less about who you sleep with and more about how you see yourself and the kind of people you choose to surround yourself with. Netflix has now brought back *The Boys in the Band* in a more contemporary New York. It feels just as challenging and true today as when the original first came out. We are definitely a complex lot but most of us wouldn't have it any other way.

GLOSSARY

acupuncture—Is a form of alternative medicine and a key component of traditional Chinese medicine in which thin needles are inserted into the body.

age of consent—The age at which an individual can legally consent to sexual activity, specifically sexual intercourse.

anabolic steroid—Sex hormone agonists, including testosterone, estrogen, and progesterone.

androgyny—A person who is ambiguous with regard to biological sex, gender identity, gender expression, or sexual identity. Or a person who has sexual traits of both sexes or neither feminine or masculine traits.

androgynous—A person who has the characteristics or nature of both male and female, or suitable to either sex, as in androgynous clothing.[1]

allosexual—The term for a person who simply experiences sexual attraction to someone. Sexual crushes or fantasies are kinds of allosexual behaviors.

animal magnetism—Attraction of one person to another based on sensory impulses, such as sight and smell.

asexual—A person who experiences an abnormally diminished sexual response to partners of both sexes.

authoritarian religion—Religion that rules instead of suggesting how people behave sexually.

balls—Is a common name for testicles.

basic sex 101—The limited information that most people begin their sex life with.

---

[1] https://www.merriam-webster.com/dictionary/androgynous.

BDSM—Is a variety of often-erotic activity or practices or role-playing involving bondage, discipline, dominance, and submission, sadomasochism, masochism, and other related behaviors.

B and D—Bondage and discipline activities involving dominant and submissive partners.

bicurious—The term for a person who is in the early stages of developing sexually and open to straight sex and bisexual sex.

bioidentical hormones—Highly effective hormones that are based on plant hormones that are engineered in the lab to be identical to human ones.

bisexual man—A man who "goes both ways," meaning that he is attracted to the opposite sex and his own sex. He may or may not actually act out on his attraction to members of his own sex.

bisexual woman—A woman who "goes both ways," because she is attracted to both the opposite sex and her own sex.

bladder—Organ that collects and contains urine before it passes from the body.

cervix—The opening at the bottom of the uterus.

chemistry—Or sexual chemistry; the sexual attraction of two people.

cisgender—A person whose sense of identity and gender corresponds to their birth sex (the opposite of transgender).

clitoris—The pleasure center of the vulva.

condoms—A common method of birth control as well as disease prevention.

cougar and cub relationships—An older woman attracts a much younger man.

cum—Sexual climax, often refers to a male.

cunnilingus—The act of oral sex on a female vulva.

cyberconnection—When two people come together online over the Internet.

cybersex—Masturbatory sex performed while interacting with another person, often performed online or over the telephone.

damaged goods—A coarse term that refers to a female who is no longer a virgin.

date rape—Sexual intercourse between a dominant (usually) male and a more submissive victim, (usually) female.

deep-throat—Oral sex with a penis until the penis is thrusting deep into the throat.

demisexual—The phenomenon of a person being attracted to another person because they have close emotional connections with that person.

depression—The clinical illness that causes psychological withdrawal and subdued mood, often experiencing prolonged sleeping.

dirty talk—Talk during sex that is intended to sexually excite the partners.

doggy style—Woman assumes the position of a dog (on hands and knees), and the male approaches from behind her.

eat pussy—Slang for cunnilingus, performing oral sex on the female vulva.

endorphins—Body chemicals that release stress and pain.

erogenous zone—The parts of the body, such as nipples, that, when touched, cause arousal.

estrogen levels—The amount of estrogen present in the body that also regulates many aspects of female development and function.

extramarital affairs—Side relationships in addition to the marital partner.

fallopian tubes—The passageway for the fertilized egg(s) to move into the uterus for gestation.

fellatio—The act of oral sex performed on the male penis.

female ejaculation—The release of liquid (as in squirting or gushing) from the vagina during sexual arousal.

fertilization—The moment that the sperm unites with the egg, creating a fertilized egg.

Fifty Shades of Grey—The book that started a new interest in sexuality involving bondage and discipline.

foreplay—Sexual games to play during sex before actual intercourse. This aspect is often overlooked, which is never a good idea.

G-spot—In addition to the clitoris, the G-spot, located just inside the vagina at the vaginal opening, is a rich source of intense orgasms.

gay lifestyle—The day-to-day existence of homosexuals as it differs from heterosexuals.

gender—Each individual has either male or female sex organs that determine gender.

gender dysphoria—An individual who is convinced he/she is trapped in a body with the wrong gender assignment.

gender fluid—Also gender nonconforming or genderqueer. Doesn't fit inside traditional male or female categories.

gender identity—How a person outwardly expresses their gender identity. Includes clothing, hairstyle, makeup, and social expressions, such as a name and pronoun choice. Examples: masculine, feminine, and androgynous. See Medscape article on gender identity.

genderqueer—An expression built around the word *queer*, to mean not aligned with heterosexual or homosexual norms.[2]

genitals—Female and male sexual body parts; also known as genitalia.

glands of the endocrine system—Regulate everything from reproduction to emotions, general health, and well-being.

heterosexual (straight) man—Is attracted to and has sex with women.

heterosexual (straight) woman—Is attracted to and has sex with men.

HIV—Human immunodeficiency virus, acquired immunodeficiency syndrome, which leads to AIDS.

hookup—Casual sex, also called one-night stand. According to Wikipedia, "a hookup culture is one that accepts and encourages casual sex encounters and other related activity, without necessarily including emotional intimacy, bonding or a committed relationship."

homophobia—Dislike of, or prejudice against, gay people.[3]

homosexual (gay) man—The term *homosexual* is considered derogatory and isn't used commonly any more. *Fag* or *faggot* are other derogatory terms. *Gay man* is the accepted term these days. *Top* and *bottom* are older terms that describe the masculine and feminine sexual roles of homosexual men.

---

[2] "What is genderqueer?" Healthline.
[3] https://en.wikipedia.org/wiki/Homophobia.

homosexual (lesbian) woman—The term *homosexual* is not considered as a proper designation and isn't used commonly inside the lesbian world. *Lesbian, gay woman,* or *gay* are all accepted terms these days. *Butch* and *fem* are older descriptive terms that describe whether a lesbian is more masculine or feminine in her appearance, sexual role, and general behavior.

hormonal levels—Changing hormonal levels are a determining factor in complicated human functions.

hormone replacement therapy—The utilization of an alternate form of hormones to replace the depleted ones.

hot flash—The sudden increase in body temperature and perspiration. Usually the face and sometimes the neck and chest are flushed red during a hot flash.

hymen—The flimsy physical "proof" that a female is still a virgin; this thin membrane surrounds the vaginal opening.

infertility—The inability of a woman to have children and of a man to impregnate a woman.

intercourse—This is the name for the most common sexual act involving the penis and the vagina.

libido—sex drive

lube—Lube, or lubricant, can be water-based or oil-based. Water-based lubricants don't degrade a condom. They are used to minimize friction during intercourse.

maidenhead—Another name for virginity.

male anatomy—The external genitalia include the penis, urethra, and scrotum.

masturbation—Self-stimulation of the genitals by both boys and girls that begins in infancy and continues into adulthood. A necessary sexual release for many people.

menopause—A physical phase in a fifty-something woman's life, after cessation of periods for a full year.

menstrual cycle—The number of days in between menstrual periods and the days of the cycle itself total approximately a month. There are twelve menstrual cycles in one year.

#MeToo—Generally women who, in the 2020s, are going public with their shameful experiences with men who accosted and/ or raped them.

metrosexual—A man who focuses heavily on grooming and fashionable dressing.

migraines—Intense and painful headaches, often attributed to tension and work pressure.

narcissistic—The name of a disorder in which the individual is basically only capable of self-love.

night sweats—The usual result of the hot flash during menopause.

old soul—An individual who is wise and mature for his/her young age.

omnisexuality—Attraction to any and all genders and sexual orientations.

orgasm—"A noun or a verb, a climax of sexual excitement, characterized by feelings of pleasure centered in the genitals and (in men) experienced as an accompaniment to ejaculation."[4]

oral sex—Includes going down, rimming, and blow jobs;[5] the act of using one's mouth (lips, tongue) to stimulate another person's sexual organ (penis or vulva), whether it is male or female.

out—An expression that means a person with a sexual orientation that is considered taboo by members of society has "come out of the closet" and shown him or herself to the world as such.

ovulation—The release of the egg(s) by the ovaries.

pansexual(ity)—Pansexuality, or omnisexuality, is the sexual, romantic, or emotional attraction toward individuals regardless of their sex or gender identity.

passive-aggressive—The traits of a person who plays emotional games with others.

pedophilia—The acts by a sexually dominant person usually over someone who is younger. Pedophiles are usually heterosexual in his or her personal sexual exploits but will make moves on people of the opposite sex during the pedophilia.

---

[4] "Orgasm," Google.
[5] https://www.avert.org/sex-stis/how-to-have-sex/oral-sex.

penis—The main exterior male genitalia that both ejaculates semen and transports urine outside the body.

period—The time during which a mature female has blood draining from the uterus because the egg(s) were not fertilized.

plenty of fish—Expression denoting plenty of potential partners or relationships.

polyamory—The practice of, or desire for, interpersonal relationships that involve physical and/or emotional intimacy with more than one partner, with the consent to engage in sexual activity of all partners involved. Polyamory is an umbrella term for nonmonogamous multipartner relationships, or nonexclusive sexual or romantic relationships.

procreation—Sex resulting in impregnation of the sexual partner with a baby, a new life.

profile—Usually refers to the personal descriptive information found on online dating sites, the profile is written to attract partners.

progesterone—Hormone released by the ovaries.

prostate gland—Found only in men, the prostate gland is located between the penis and the rectum. It produces fluid that helps to make up semen.[6]

protection—A condom and a dental dam to protect against HIV and STDs.

puberty—The intense period of sexual development in a young person who is leaving childhood and entering adulthood.

pussy—Slang for female sex organ.

queer—Nonconformist to traditional norms of gender or sexuality, usually refers to male homosexual but also as a general term.

questioning (sexually)—A person whose sexual orientation is in a state of flux and willingness to try out different partners, which may result in a change of orientation in the future.

raison d'être—French for the reason to exist, or purpose.

rape—The act of sexually forcing oneself on another person for sexual intercourse.

---

[6] www.prostatecancerfree.com.

restore the hymen—A surgical procedure to create a blockage which will bleed when ruptured by intercourse.

rimming—Giving pleasure to a person's anus with mouth, tongue, hand, or object.

safe sex—Practicing safe sex does not include unprotected oral sex; sex protected with condoms and dental dams to prevent HIV and STDs.

sapiophile or sapiosexual—Individual whose attraction to another person is based on their intelligence, which is the major turn on.

scrotum—The testicles and the sac that contains them.

selflessness—One of the three essential ingredients to successfully pleasuring your partner. The other two are communication and oral sex. If you can be much more selfless, your entire approach to sex will be different.

sex life—The sexual experiences of an individual add up to his/her sex life.

sex play—This is what sexuality is called when it isn't for procreation but for fun and relaxation together.

sexual attractiveness—The attraction of one person to another based on nonverbal qualities, such as expression, scent, a pout, and much more.

sexual desire—The attraction of one person to another for the many purpose of having sex.

sexual incompatibility—When one person is turned off to another person.

sexual infidelity—Cheating on partner or spouse with another sexual partner.

sexual orientation—A person's general physical, romantic, and emotional attraction to another person.

sexual personality—What is your sexuality like? Find out with online tests on page 41.

sexual repression—Exterior means of diminishing sexual expression, often by one's culture.

sexual tension—The tension that builds up between sexual acts and release with orgasm.

sexually compatible—Two people who are sexually attracted to each other. This is seldom clear until the two have met and spent at least some time together.

sex drive—The frequency and degree that a person wishes to engage in sexual activities.

sex reassignment surgery—The process involved in a transgender person's change from male to female or female to male. Referred to as top and bottom surgeries.

social or religion-induced guilt—Guilt that is suffered because of society or religion.

STDs—Sexually transmitted diseases that include syphilis, gonorrhea, chlamydia, and herpes.

straight—The sexual urges of a straight (heterosexual) person is for members of the opposite sex.

sucking cock—The vulgar term for fellatio, which is the sucking of the male organ for the purpose of bringing on an orgasm.

sugar daddy—Usually a much older man who financially cares for someone, usually much younger.

sugar mama—Usually a much older female who financially cares for someone, usually much younger.

taboo—Any practice that would be too embarrassing to tell others that you did.

testes—These are the testicles that contain sperm.

testosterone—The primary male sex hormone produced in the testicles. The female also produces testosterone in her ovaries and adrenal system.

tranny—[7] Often meant as a derogatory term for a transgender, transsexual, transvestite, or cross-dresser.

transgender—A gender identity, also transsexual. A person who identifies as the opposite sex from the gender assigned at birth. A transgender person may have surgery or not and may be attracted to the same sex or the opposite sex. A transgender individual may be attracted to those who identify as straight, homosexual (lesbians or gay men), bisexual, or queer.

---

[7] Wikipedia.

transsexual—See transgender.

transvestite—Dressing up in elaborate often sexy clothing of the opposite sex and often appearing in public places in order to be seen. According to popular understanding about it, this group is comprised mainly by heterosexual men, who can have "normal" relationships with their female partner, who is very understanding and supportive. Or he can act out his cross-dressing rituals in secret. Or they could become a famous gay cross-dresser named Ru Paul. It's important to stress that individuals who are asexual, bisexual, heterosexual, or homosexual are all candidates for cross-dressing.

uterus—The part of the female's body that contains the fetus during gestation. The uterus opens into the vagina.

vagina—The passageway from the female exterior sexual organ, the vulva, into the interior (cervix, uterus, and sexual organs for procreation).

vaginal orgasms—Orgasms that originate inside the vagina, usually stimulated only by the penis during intercourse.

vulva—The exterior of the main female sexual organ.

virginity—The physical state a female is in before penetrative sex.

wedding-night virginity testing—Inspection of the sheet for hymen blood after the first intercourse to prove that a female is a virgin.

ABOUT THE AUTHOR

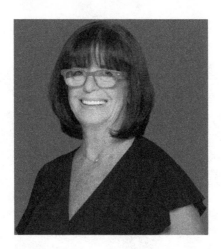

Pamela Hepburn Fisk is not a specialist in human sexuality. However, she has well-developed ideas about what is missing from many relationships; she is a very sexual person and a professional writer, and therefore she presents herself as qualified to author this book called *A Complete Guide to Pleasuring Your Partner: The Sex Education You Never Got.* The reaction to the book has been so overwhelmingly positive that she realized her dream of writing it and getting it published were both entirely realistic. Originally from Massachusetts, Ms. Fisk attended New York University Film School with a particular emphasis on dramatic writing, which prepared her for a twenty-five-year copywriting career, after which she retired and began research for two books that she planned to write. The first one, about politics, never came to fruition; and the second, about sex, resulted in this work, which she hopes will entertain and educate her readers in entirely new ways of expressing themselves in the bedroom.

CPSIA information can be obtained
at www.ICGtesting.com
Printed in the USA
BVHW031821211221
624510BV00025B/59